Another excellent book on IB.
by a patient with specialist
questions raised by every patie
summarising the evidence in a 1
recommended.

MU00780275

Professor Simon Travis, FRCP, Professor of Clinical Gastroenterology, University of Oxford, UK. Former President of the European Crohn's & Colitis Organisation (ECCO)

This book is a must read for any IBD patient seeking guidance on how to be resilient in the face of an inflammatory bowel disease diagnosis. Dr Mikocka-Walus, a health psychologist, behavioral scientist and IBD patient herself, conveys the best scientific evidence available on the holistic care of IBD in a very accessible and engaging way. I will be recommending this to all of my patients and families in the USA.

Associate Professor Laurie Keefer, PhD, GI Psychologist, Director of Psychobehavioral Research. Susan and Leonard Feinstein IBD Clinical Center, Mount Sinai Hospital, NYC, USA

Dr Mikocka-Walus has provided a comprehensive and reader friendly IBD resource, translating complex information and clinical research about the disease into everyday language. Her matter-of-fact discussion about all aspects of living with IBD, from stools to stress to sexuality, is not only informative, uniquely blending science and personal journey, but will be reassuring for those with IBD and their families.

Professor Lesley Graff, Head, Department of Clinical Health Psychology, Max Rady College of Medicine, University of Manitoba & Medical Director, Clinical Health Psychology Program, Winnipeg Regional Health Authority, Manitoba CANADA

Dr Mikocka-Walus delivers a cogent review of inflammatory bowel disease from a unique perspective: that of a health professional who suffers from the disease. **IBD and the Gut-Brain Connection** *provides an insightful summary of life with IBD, with a particular focus on the impact of mood on disease outcomes, and how this can be managed. The text is a valuable additional information source to patients with IBD, and is highly recommended.*

Dr David Gracie, BSc MB ChB MRCP, Gastroenterology specialist trainee, Bradford Royal Infirmary, UK

To my parents, Basia and Tomek, with love

Illness is the night side of life, a more onerous citizenship. Everyone who is born holds dual citizenship, in the kingdom of the well and in the kingdom of the sick. Although we all prefer to use the good passport, sooner or later each of us is obliged, at least for a spell, to identify ourselves as citizens of that other place.

Susan Sontag, Illness as Metaphor

Nobody realises that some people expend tremendous energy merely to be normal.

Albert Camus, Notebooks: 1942–1951

IBD and the Gut–Brain Connection

A patient and carer's guide to
taming Crohn's disease
and ulcerative colitis

Dr Antonina Mikocka-Walus

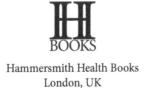

Hammersmith Health Books
London, UK

First published in 2018 by Hammersmith Health Books – an imprint of
Hammersmith Books Limited
4/4A Bloomsbury Square, London WC1A 2RP, UK
www.hammersmithbooks.co.uk

© 2018, Dr Antonina Mikocka-Walus

Disclaimer: The information in this book is of a general nature
and is meant for educational purposes only. It is not intended as
medical advice. The contents may not be used to treat, or diagnose,
any particular disease or any particular person. Applying elements
from this publication does not constitute a professional relationship
or professional advice or services. No endorsement or warranty is
explicitly given or implied by any entity connected to this content.

As always, if you have pre-existing health issues and especially if
you are taking any medications, you are advised first to consult your
health practitioner before making any changes to your lifestyle and
diet.

British Library Cataloguing in Publication Data: a CIP record of this
book is available from the British Library.

Print ISBN: 978-1-78161-140-1
Ebook ISBN: 978-1-78161-141-8

Editor: Georgina Bentliff
Cover design: Sylvia Kwan
Text designed and typeset by: Julie Bennett, Bespoke Publishing Ltd
Index: Dr Laurence Errington
Production: Helen Whitehorn of Path Projects Ltd
Printed and bound by: TJ International Ltd, UK

Contents

Contents

Contents

Foreword

The question is not how to get cured, but how to live.

Joseph Conrad, *Lord Jim*

Over five million people worldwide battle inflammatory bowel disease (IBD) every day – an invisible, debilitating illness that burdens its suffers with a lifelong struggle.

As CEO of Crohn's & Colitis Australia (the peak national body representing IBD sufferers nationwide), I have seen firsthand how frightened people recently diagnosed or living with IBD can be. Time and again, IBD sufferers are confused by their diagnosis, worried that IBD will severely affect their day-to-day lives, and afraid that their dreams are unattainable. With IBD patients stigmatised and generally misunderstood, they can even be embarrassed to discuss their illness with family, friends and co-workers.

That's precisely where this book comes in. As an IBD sufferer and health professional herself, Antonina's book is a window into what life is really like when you suffer from a chronic illness. With a lovely blend of gentle humour interspersed by scientific fact and personal experience, Antonina answers so many of the questions that recently diagnosed IBD patients want to ask but are hesitant to voice.

So often, IBD patients struggle to grasp all that is happening in the medicine and science of their illness. This book explains all this in simple, readily accessible terms. It delves into the psychological impact of IBD, as well as what to expect from medical treatments and therapies, presenting a refreshingly unique holistic approach to IBD care. Antonina's personal experiences will resonate with IBD patients, making them feel heard. It will make them feel as though their emotional, physical and mental concerns are shared – they will understand that they're not alone.

A book like this matters because it teaches IBD patients, along with their loved ones, how to live with an illness that is both challenging and invisible. It teaches us to work together to overcome fear and embarrassment, and to tackle the unknown. Thank you, Antonina, for sharing your vast knowledge and your personal story that may help other IBD patients feel more 'normal'.

Whether you've been recently diagnosed with IBD yourself, or your partner, sister, brother, mother, father or best friend suffers from IBD, within the pages of this book you will discover deep insights into what it is really like to live with this crazy, chronic illness.

Francesca Manglaviti
Chief Executive Officer
Crohn's & Colitis Australia

Acknowledgements

I've carried this book in me for years. I have penned tens of scientific articles and communications for other health professionals but have never written anything dedicated 100% to my fellow IBD sufferers. My huge thanks to all those who have helped me in bringing this project to fruition.

Particular thanks are due to Dr Simon Knowles and Dr Cate Howell – excellent scientists, health practitioners and fantastic colleagues who provided comments on the book's drafts. Huge thanks to my beta-readers: Elizabeth Enticott and Bruce James.

To my publisher, Georgina Bentliff, for believing in this book and to Carolyn White, my editor, for making the book what it is today.

To my family: my siblings Jula and Antek, my aunts Katarzyna and Ewa and uncles Andrzej and Mirek and my cousins Ola and Pakis, and to my faithful high school friends who were by my side when I needed them most: Karo, Wiola, Aga, Justa, Dano and Mariusz – this would have been so much harder without you.

To my husband, Bart, special thanks for having the patience to share a life with someone addicted to toilet spotting.

To my aunt, Dr Bożena Dębska, an excellent doctor who saved me years of misdiagnosis. Thank you for all the years of supporting my family and me in our IBD adventure.

About the author

Antonina Mikocka-Walnus is Associate Professor in Health Psychology at Deakin University, Australia; Visiting Associate Professor in Psychology at the University of Adelaide, Australia; and Visiting Senior Research Fellow at the University of York, UK. Dr Antonina Mikocka-Walus is a psychologist, health scientist and writer interested in IBD, a condition that has been her intimate companion since adolescence. She was born and raised in Warsaw, Poland and emigrated to Australia in her mid-twenties. She completed her Masters in psychology at the University of Warsaw and her doctoral studies in medicine at the University of Adelaide and has since worked in several Australian and British universities. The main theme of her research has been the psychology of IBD. She has conducted studies examining the relationship between anxiety and depression and disease activity in IBD, the role of psychotherapy and antidepressants in IBD, and patients' and doctors' views on the psychology of IBD. She has contributed to the international guidelines on IBD care. Her research has led to changes in how IBD services operate, with her recommendations for the use of an integrated model of care now being implemented in several clinics worldwide, including Australia, Europe and South America. She has published widely, with over 90 books, book chapters and research papers, and has received multiple research grants to fund her studies in IBD.

She lives in Melbourne, Australia with her talented husband, composer Bart Walus.

Preface

There are different kinds of poo. A normal poo is a perfect compromise between softness and firmness. It is not liquid; neither should it be lumpy or hard to pass. Picture a soft sausage or one with gentle cracks marking its surface.

I am not saying what an ideal poo should look like based on my own experience. After spending most of my life living with inflammatory bowel disease (IBD), I am no longer certain what is normal when it comes to poo. I need to consult external sources, such as the Bristol Stool Scale.[1] This tells me that the familiar mushy wastes I frequently flush in my toilet are a sign of inflammation and that, for most people, this is not something they are used to seeing in their toilet bowl.

You may take me for a poo purist, choosing one type of poo and discriminating against all others. Surely people vary, so should their poo? Well, people may see differently shaped poo being flashed down their toilets, but it is very clear to any health professional with expertise in treating people's guts that chronic diarrhoea is a sign of a disorder, as is constipation.

There are many conditions that may cause changed patterns in your bowel movements, but the aim of this book is not to help you self-diagnose or tell you about them all. This is a book about IBD and addressed to anyone who already has their IBD diagnosis or who knows or cares for someone living with IBD.

Why should I be the one telling you about IBD?

I am a patient and have lived with IBD for over 20 years. I experience the symptoms if not daily then at least weekly. I have had numerous medical treatments and medical procedures. I know at first hand how tormenting the pain can be. For many, it is both literally and figuratively a pain in the butt, and because the rectum is full of nerve endings, it really hurts.

I have also often felt ashamed of my IBD symptoms. I have interrupted family outings with constant toilet spotting. I have blushed under the scornful looks of people who believed I had no right to use a disabled toilet because I appeared too healthy. I have struggled with fatigue as a result of my IBD and I have noticed its impact on my mood.

I started being ill in my teens and thus I have experienced both paediatric and adult IBD care. I am a daughter, a wife and a friend – I know what impact IBD may have on social interactions, on the decision to start a family. I am an employee, and was a student for many years, so I know that IBD impacts on educational and career prospects. I have used health services in several countries and understand how health professionals interact with patients. I have sat on patient panels and advised patient organisations.

As IBD significantly changed the way I live and perceived the world from an early age, I decided to get to know it. After all, with no cure on the horizon, we will most likely be mates till I die, so why not? Initially, I merely had a selfish hope to make my own life better. But as I immersed myself in studying psychology, and later medicine, and as I got to know many people struggling with IBD, my life's goal shifted from the self-centred search for a cure to sharing what I learnt with fellow sufferers, their families and friends.

Professionally, I wear several pairs of shoes. (I prefer this expression to wearing hats, as hats are not really my kind of thing, and shoes ... well they are a lifelong passion.) I am a psychologist and a health scientist. I have worked as a practising psychologist, researcher and teacher, and my career has focused on developing ways to better manage IBD. I promote knowledge of the complexity of IBD among psychology, medical and nursing students, with the hope that when they meet a patient suffering from IBD they will be able to treat them holistically, rather than focusing merely on the bowel. I am also a writer. I love both science and creative writing and a lot of what I write is dedicated to IBD. The more I write and talk about this complex disease, the more I understand it, so I intend to keep going.

What are the effects of my work? I have helped quite a few patients through my psychotherapy work. The first time a patient told me she wouldn't be here if it had not been for me, I knew all the effort I had put into getting an education and specialist training was worth it, even though my IBD got crazy around examination sessions, and I always hated taking exams for fear I would have to run to the loo in the middle of them. I have taught hundreds of students and have published a large number of research papers, book chapters and other science papers (search for my name in Google Scholar, for example, to see my research work on IBD). While I haven't found the cure, I have contributed to improved understanding of IBD and its treatment.

IBD research

At the moment, hundreds of scientists around the world are toiling towards finding the cure for IBD. It's a slow and often disheartening process as IBD research is not well funded. Although studies show that IBD is associated with a huge personal and societal burden and large healthcare costs, its relatively low incidence (i.e. how often it occurs), compared with other chronic conditions, such as diabetes or cardiovascular disease, means research funders prioritise these other conditions. On one hand, that's understandable. People die more commonly from heart problems than from IBD. But IBD patients on average suffer their symptoms for a much longer time. The peak incidence is in the twenties, and with more and more children getting sick, the incidence shifts towards a younger age and more severe disease presentation. We thus suffer for decades and while we may not die of IBD, it makes our lives miserable, often on a daily basis, limiting our educational and occupational chances and significantly affecting our family and social lives.

IBD also makes people more prone to other conditions. For example, people with IBD have a greater risk of developing arthritis, asthma and bronchitis than other members of the population. Those with ulcerative colitis, one of IBD's subtypes, also have an increased risk of chronic renal disease and multiple sclerosis.

There are no easy answers when it comes to cure. Like cancer, IBD is a complex condition. While we know that the environment, our genes and our immune system play a role, we are still not certain what IBD's aetiology (i.e. cause) actually is. We may need to wait decades before IBD becomes curable, but in the meantime the treatment becomes more effective and safer. I think of myself as fortunate living at the time when there is such a variety of IBD treatments on the market. The last 20 years have made a huge difference to how IBD is treated. Most patients have access to biologics, a novel IBD treatment I will tell you more about in Chapter 9. IBD can now be controlled in most cases through using either medication or surgery. Of course, it comes and goes as it wishes but at least we know what to do when it flares.

In this book, I will tell you what IBD is, how it is currently treated and what the typical problems associated with the disease are. I will discuss the issues which many patients wonder about: the role of stress in IBD; IBD in children and adolescent populations and the elderly; pregnancy, fertility and sexuality; fatigue; mental health; drug treatment and surgery; diet; psychotherapy and hypnotherapy; antidepressants and holistic care.

I will share with you my own perspective when I can but will also provide an overview of what science tells us on each topic. I will largely rely on the sources called systematic reviews (unless these are unavailable and then I will report on results of the best quality single studies).

In science, to improve our certainty that one treatment works better than another, or better than a placebo (a dummy tablet), systematic reviews are conducted. These reviews combine other studies using a well-defined methodology and, by critiquing these single studies, provide a more objective recommendation than would come from one study only. Some of these reviews also combine the results of previous studies using a statistical technique called a meta-analysis. To put it simply, imagine that you are aware of 10 different studies examining acupuncture in IBD. Some of these studies are small but a few are quite large, with several thousands of participants. Some are conducted using well-described and replicable methodologies while others report poorly on their method or results. Systematic reviews can combine the results of all these individual studies and make the reader aware which of them could be trusted more than others. The outcome of such a review could be a recommendation for practice. You may like to visit the Cochrane Library (http:// www.cochranelibrary.com/) which is a home to some excellent systematic reviews. You can read their summaries free of charge and keep up to date with current evidence on IBD care.

While science-based, this book is meant to be a resource for patients, their families and friends. It is not meant as a text for health professionals. Medical practitioners interested in the holistic approach to IBD which I describe here, may like to read a scientific book I have co-edited with another IBD psychologist, Dr Simon Knowles.[2] However, references are provided for each chapter of this book for those readers interested in scientific sources.

I hope you find my personal observations, my professional

experience, and my view on what science on IBD tells us useful. My wish is that this book may improve your knowledge of IBD. Known evil is better than unfamiliar evil. I have noticed that the more I understand about IBD, the easier it becomes to manage and live with it. I hope it will be the same for you.

Dr Antonina Mikocka-Walus
2018

Part I

Understanding IBD

Chapter 1

What is IBD?

The name 'inflammatory bowel disease' tells you that IBD is a disease of the intestines – that is, of the small and/or large bowel – and that some reddening and swelling must be involved, as these are the signs of inflammation. In IBD, our tummy (also called the abdomen) hurts mostly around and below the navel area where the intestines are located, though in some people upper tummy pain also occurs, and often diarrhoea, bleeding and nausea. However, explaining IBD as a condition is not as simple as this. Let's first focus on what healthy digestion is.

When we place food in our mouth we start the process of digestion, whereby food is changed into energy and nutrients to feed the body. The food passes down a long duct, our gastrointestinal tract, beginning in the mouth and leading through the oesophagus, into the stomach and then first to the small, and later to the large intestine (they are also called small and large bowel, respectively). The final portion of the large intestine is the rectum, which ends with the anus where the wastes of the digestive process (i.e. stool, popularly called poo) are discharged.

Each section of the gastrointestinal tract has its part to play in digestion. The small bowel absorbs 90% of nutrients from the food we have eaten. The large bowel absorbs water from what is left after digestion, and expels the solid wastes via the rectum and anus from the body. When inflammation and ulcers appear in the small or large bowel, the bowel stops working as it should – we no longer absorb all the necessary nutrients, minerals and water, and we notice unpleasant symptoms such as diarrhoea, bleeding and pain, which don't go away after a few days as they would if this was a simple bout of gastroenteritis. This is usually when we visit a doctor, and, after some investigations, we may learn that we have inflammatory bowel disease. But what exactly IBD is, is not yet fully understood. Let me briefly show you how the thinking on IBD has evolved throughout history and what is currently believed to cause it.

The history of IBD

IBD has been around for a long time. There are historical reviews indicating that the ancient Greeks and Chinese described cases of abdominal pain and diarrhoea that resembled IBD.[1] IBD has two main subtypes: Crohn's disease (CD) and ulcerative colitis (UC). The term 'ulcerative colitis' was first used to describe the disorder by a British pathologist, Samuel Wilks, in 1859.[2] Crohn's disease was not officially named until 1932, when Burrill Crohn wrote of the discovery of a new intestinal disease, 'terminal (regional) ileitis', in a letter to the American Gastroenterological Association. To honour the discoverer, surgeon Brian Brooke renamed the disease, and the term 'Crohn's disease' entered common use.

In the 1930s and 1940s, a view predominated that psychological problems played a central role in the development of ulcerative colitis. Sigmund Freud's work (on 'talk therapy') was influential at the time, so this wasn't surprising, and there were some documented cases of UC being successfully treated or managed with psychotherapy. In addition, the physiologists of this era – for example, Walter Cannon, famous for his research on stress – also believed that emotional calmness was important to normal digestion, hence the thinking that psychological distress equals poor digestion.

We now know that this view is not completely wrong – stress plays an important part in IBD as I will explain in Chapter 2 where I provide an overview of the gut-brain links and their implications for those living with IBD. However, the spread of research into physiology, immunity and genetics in the second half of the twentieth century meant that IBD started to be considered as a physiological condition rather than a psychological one (that is, to do with the functioning of the body rather than the mind). In 1969, colonoscopy – a procedure where a tube is inserted into the rectum and a little camera is passed up to observe the inside of the bowel – was introduced and it allowed doctors to see inflammatory changes in the bowel for the first time.

Modern theories on the causes of IBD

Later studies into immunity have proposed that IBD develops when our bodies struggle to tolerate the bacteria inhabiting our gut.[3] Genetics has also contributed to our understanding of the disease. IBD occurs in people who are genetically predisposed to getting it – there are more than 100 distinct changes to the genes that are present in people living with IBD.[4] There is also an increased risk of IBD among family members of patients with IBD (stronger for those with CD than UC) and particularly in siblings. The earlier the onset of IBD, the stronger the genetic link and the higher risk for the family members.

The environment has long been considered an important factor in IBD's causation. There is a well-known theory on how IBD came about, called the 'hygiene hypothesis'. It states that conditions such as IBD are common nowadays because we have little contact with bacteria during our childhood.[5] The cleaner we become, the more sanitised our childhoods, the more prone we become to inflammatory conditions later in life. Studies on environmental factors show that IBD is more common in industrialised countries and in urban societies and in people with fewer siblings and generally smaller families.[6,7]

There are also other factors contributing to its incidence.

- Smoking, for example, makes one more likely to develop CD,[6] though it doesn't have this effect on UC.

- Studies have also shown that some diets make IBD more likely. A high consumption of sugars and fats has been associated with an increased risk of developing IBD,[8,9] while high intake of dietary fibre, including fruit and vegetable consumption, may protect against IBD.[6] It is important to note that this evidence doesn't tell us what we should eat when we have IBD. Instead, it simply says that people who were diagnosed with IBD could have been eating this diet before the diagnosis and it may have contributed (together with other factors) to their IBD coming about. I will tell you more about diet for IBD in Chapter 11.

- Prolonged use of the oral contraceptive pill is another factor which may make IBD more likely to occur. Hormones used in the pill have an impact on inflammatory processes in the body.[6]

- A protective factor is the removal of your appendix (a tiny sac attached to the large bowel). Those without an appendix have a lower risk of developing UC. The relationship is, however, less clear for CD.[6]

- Breastfeeding is a protective factor, with those breastfed in childhood less likely to develop IBD.[6]

- On the other hand, taking repeated courses of antibiotics in early childhood is another risk factor for the development of IBD.[5]

- Similarly, frequent use of nonsteroidal anti-inflammatory drugs, e.g. ibuprofen or aspirin, is a predisposing factor for IBD.[6]

What do all these studies tell us about the causes of IBD? They tell us that IBD is a disease in which the immune system reacts in an exaggerated way to normal bacteria inhabiting the intestines, a response which may be triggered by environmental factors, or come about because someone has a genetic predisposition.

Types of IBD

The two main types of IBD are Crohn's disease and ulcerative colitis, but there is also a third type, indeterminate colitis (IC). This term is used when the disease resembles both CD and UC and neither can be clearly distinguished. A minority of patients (approximately 10%) fit into this category. In research studies, IC is often combined with UC because it resembles it more than the CD.

I am one of those few patients who have suffered from all three types of IBD. When I was diagnosed with IBD, it presented as Crohn's disease and it was CD for as long as I lived in Poland. My symptoms then included diarrhoea, weight loss, occasional tummy pain, fever and anaemia.

When I emigrated to Australia, something strange started happening to my body. First, the disease went completely quiet for a few years. I guessed this must have been due to the change in climate and diet. In Australia, I stopped eating as much meat as I had been used to in Poland and switched to seafood and vegetables. I also consumed less dairy. During the long hot summers my body craved a different kind of nourishment. But after a few years, IBD returned in a changed form. My symptoms shifted to rectal pain and bleeding. I no longer lost weight – in fact, I put on weight – but my diarrhoea remained the same. After a colonoscopy, I was given a new diagnosis of ulcerative colitis. My treatment changed as well, as the disease was now located much lower (in the rectum, so at the end of the large bowel) and enemas (a medication in a liquid form provided through the rectum) became more effective than steroids taken orally.

When I moved to the UK, the disease went silent as it had for a few years after my first emigration to Australia, though not completely this time. I had to use the enemas regularly, every few weeks, whereas in the past I had enjoyed long periods of remission. I was never completely free of symptoms, but on the other hand they were never unbearable. After another series of investigations, I was told I now had indeterminate colitis. The treatment remained the same as for UC.

I am now back in Australia and watch my body with interest. Which of the old friends will it be this time?

Typical symptoms of IBD

What is common for all three types of IBD is that some people have severe symptoms while others only suffer occasionally. The cycles of remission (quiescent disease when people are symptom-free or have limited symptoms only) and flares (active disease, with the full spectrum of symptoms) also vary. Some people can be free of symptoms (in remission) for years while others may have just days or weeks of freedom and very lengthy flares.

Crohn's disease

CD is characterised by inflammation anywhere in the digestive system (from the mouth to the anus), but most commonly in the last section of the small intestine or in the colon (i.e. the large intestine).

In CD, the typical symptoms are: recurring diarrhoea; abdominal pain and cramping (worse after meals); fatigue (i.e. extreme tiredness); weight loss; and mucus (and sometimes also blood) in stools. Less commonly, people report a high temperature (of over 38°C); nausea; vomiting; and so-called 'extra-intestinal' (outside the intestine) symptoms, such as: joint pain and swelling; uveitis (inflammation of an eye); inflammation of the skin, presenting as painful, red and swollen patches, most typically on the legs; and mouth ulcers also called 'aphthae'.

Ulcerative colitis

In UC, the colon and rectum become inflamed. When you observe the bowel through a camera during a colonoscopy, small ulcers may be noticed which bleed and produce pus.

The symptoms of UC include recurring diarrhoea which may contain blood, mucus or pus; abdominal pain; and urgency (feeling that you need to empty your bowel immediately). Fatigue is also present, though its levels are slightly lower than in CD. Loss of appetite and weight loss do occur in some people as do the extra-intestinal symptoms described above for CD. In severe cases, with many bowel movements a day, shortness of breath; a fast or irregular heartbeat; fever; and blood in stools becoming more pronounced can also happen.

Indeterminate colitis

IC, as mentioned above, may have overlapping symptoms of both CD and UC and is usually treated similarly to UC. You can ask why it matters that we know whether we have UC or IC if the treatment for both is the same. The answer is, there are important differences if surgery such as colectomy (removal of the bowel) is required. Patients with UC usually respond better to it than those with IC who, on the other hand, respond better than those with CD. Thus, in the case of planned surgery, it's important to be sure which disease type you have.

How common is IBD?

When IBD was first described and named, it was a rare disease which few people had heard about. It owes its wider recognition to American President Dwight Eisenhower who suffered bowel symptoms for years but was only diagnosed with CD in his sixties. He had to undergo emergency surgery for CD and spoke about it openly, thus promoting understanding of IBD among the general public.

IBD occurrence increased in the developed countries in the second half of the twentieth century, and it is now increasing in developing countries. According to recent studies, between 300 and 480 people per 100,000 are affected by IBD in western countries.

Over 5 million people now live with IBD around the world. There are currently 2.5–3 million people with the condition in Europe, 1.4 million people in the US, 233,000 in Canada, and over 75,000 in Australia. In the developed countries, CD is more common than UC, whereas the trend is reversed in Asia. There is quite a significant geographic difference in IBD's incidence between eastern, western, northern and southern countries. The overall annual IBD occurrence in western Europe is roughly twice as high as the rates in eastern Europe. Similarly, the frequency of UC is 40% and CD 80% higher in the north of Europe as compared with the south.

IBD affects both males and females, but it's slightly more common in males (the rate for males is 56% as compared with 44% in females). It is most common in the 20–29 years age group, in populations with high socio-economic status, and those of Jewish ancestry, and uncommon in indigenous populations (those who have lived in a place for centuries before modern times and live in distinct traditional ways).

In terms of how IBD behaves, we know it is a recurring condition, but how often does it recur? During a period of two years of observation, approximately 50% of UC patients are likely to be in remission but the chance of a flare in five years is high – approximately 80%.

In CD, 34% of people flare after one year of observation, 70% after five years, and 77% after 10 years of observation. While the majority of IBD patients experience both remissions and flares / relapses, 20–25% of patients have continuous symptoms, so they are never in remission. Note that these rates come from studies that may have started quite a long time ago when biologics (see Chapter 9) were not widely available, and thus the course of IBD over time may improve in the future as we get better treatment. For example, current hospitalisation rates in CD are quite high, with 50% of European CD patients needing a hospital stay within 10 years from diagnosis, but these rates are dropping. Moreover, although 30–50% of CD patients require surgery in the 10 years following diagnosis, these rates are also falling. In contrast, just 10% of UC patients presently require colectomy (major bowel surgery) within 10 years of their diagnosis. Extra-intestinal manifestations are present in up to 40% of CD patients and up to 20% of UC patients.

Conditions that coexist with IBD

I mentioned in the Preface to this book that IBD is associated with a greater likelihood of suffering from other inflammatory conditions, such as asthma or arthritis. What is, however, more common than these inflammatory 'comorbidities', is an overlap of IBD with irritable bowel syndrome (IBS). Another common issue is fatigue. Cancer is a fear often reported by those living with IBD, and although cancer is a less common comorbidity than IBS or fatigue, the risk needs to be addressed and understood.

Irritable bowel syndrome and IBD

IBS is commonly confused with IBD, as they have similar names and symptoms. But IBS differs from IBD. It does not cause ulcers or lesions and when a patient undergoes a colonoscopy, no clear signs of disease can be spotted in the bowel, though the patient reports aggravating symptoms of diarrhoea and / or constipation, pain, cramping and bloating. The pain or discomfort is generally relieved after a bowel movement.

In the case of IBD, IBS may appear during periods of remission. In such cases, patients continue to report diarrhoea and pain even though the common inflammation markers are within the normal range and colonoscopy shows that they are in remission. In fact, 40% of IBD patients report symptoms consistent with IBS and we are four times more likely to have IBS than the rest of the population.[10] What is more, 50% of first-degree relatives of people who suffer IBD report symptoms of IBS, meaning the two can be genetically linked.[11] Some current research suggests that IBS in IBD may be a product of inflammation which is not detected by the standard inflammation tests, but this needs to be further investigated.

Interestingly, patients with IBS in IBD have higher levels of anxiety and depression than other IBD patients. IBS is, in fact, a condition serving as a model for the importance of gut-brain interactions, with a recent study showing that people who have anxiety and depression and no bowel problems tend to develop gastrointestinal symptoms over time, while those with bowel problems and no anxiety or depression initially, over time are at a higher risk of developing these common mental disorders.[11A] It is therefore not surprising that psychological factors such as anxiety may contribute to having IBS in IBD[10] and that counselling and psychotherapy are recommended in people having this comorbidity. Antidepressants and dietary interventions are other treatments commonly used. The latter often entails a low FODMAP diet (a diet restricting some carbohydrates – see page 112) or a diet addressing fructose malabsorption, which is common in CD. I discuss diet in IBD in Chapter 11.

Fatigue

Fatigue (i.e. sense of tiredness or weakness) is common even in healthy humans. Its purpose is to prevent injury when our body is no longer functioning optimally. When we are sick, fatigue makes us rest so that the body can heal itself. Unfortunately, in chronic illnesses the same mechanism, of making us feel tired so we can get better, doesn't work. Fatigue becomes chronic – IBD can't be cured after all, yet the body unsuccessfully tries. Even when we get effective treatment, such as biologics (see page 90), fatigue remains.

We can feel physically fatigued (we can't physically perform), cognitively fatigued (our thinking is clouded) or psychologically fatigued (we lack motivation and have a low mood). We can develop all these types of fatigue or just one or two.

Fatigue is very common in IBD and is associated with poorer quality of life and 'comorbid mood disorders' – anxiety and depression. It is linked to inflammation, poor sleep and psychological problems.

Disease activity (inflammation) doesn't explain fatigue completely, as many patients in remission also suffer fatigue, but it explains to some degree why those flaring their IBD have higher rates of fatigue than those in remission. IBD patients often report problems sleeping, and poor sleep has been linked to disease activity in IBD. Fatigue is associated with psychological problems, such as depression, but it can also exist without psychological disorders. There are numerous other reasons for fatigue in IBD – for example, malnutrition and deficiencies of iron, vitamin D3, magnesium or B-group vitamins.

Treatment of fatigue starts with adjustment of IBD medication to ensure inflammation is addressed in the first instance. Currently taken medication is screened and the ones which can contribute to fatigue are stopped. Vitamin supplementation may also be added. Lifestyle changes can be recommended, such as increased physical activity, better sleep 'hygiene' (addressing factors that are detrimental to sleep) and diet. Psychotherapies such as CBT (discussed in Chapter 12) are also useful for fatigue.[12]

Cancer

IBD patients often worry about developing cancer and overestimate its risk but receive little reassuring information from their doctors about this. While the risk of having colorectal cancer *is* increased in IBD, in recent years due to routine colonoscopies and good maintenance therapy (5ASA drugs) it is decreasing.[13] As IBD patients are monitored for it regularly, cancer can be detected early, when it is still treatable. Thus, while we are as a group at risk of it, only a small percentage of IBD patients develop colorectal cancer.

Specifically, in UC, approximately 1.6% of patients will develop colorectal cancer during 14 years of follow-up.[14] In CD, 5.6% of patients develop colorectal cancer during 30 years of follow-up.[15]

Which IBD patients are most likely to develop colorectal cancer? Those with:

- a long history of colitis
- extensive inflammation in the colon
- coexistent primary sclerosis cholangitis (a disease of a liver)
- a family history of colorectal cancer
- colonic strictures (narrowing of the intestines)
- multiple polyps
- folic acid (vitamin B9) deficiencies
- and those not taking IBD medications or
- not receiving adequate surveillance (e.g. not getting regular colonoscopies).[16]

What can you do to minimise your colorectal cancer risk? If you don't take any maintenance therapy (such as 5ASA) or haven't had a colonoscopy for over three years, it may be worth speaking with your doctor. You should take maintenance therapy for IBD all the time (it reduces the risk of colorectal cancer[16]) and colonoscopies need to be scheduled every few years (exactly when depends on your disease; for some people it needs to be as often as annually). Similarly, if your folic acid levels are low, supplementation may be needed. Eat a healthy diet and do some exercise (see Chapter 11) – these two recommendations are universal for all people, not just IBD patients.

What about the risk of other cancers? We know that some IBD medications, such as thiopurines and biologics, may increase the risk of developing cancer (e.g. lymphoma) but this risk is very low (much lower than for colorectal cancer)[17] and thus the benefits of these medications outweigh the risk.

Can you die of IBD?

I only asked myself this question a few years ago. I'm not sure why I never thought of it before. Perhaps because I was diagnosed at the age when one seems to be immortal or perhaps I simply didn't want to think about it? I decided to look into it properly while writing this book.

Reading through current research I learnt that in most cases IBD is not a terminal illness. In UC, the mortality is comparable to the general population. The risk of mortality is, however, increased in CD.[18-20]

For both CD and UC, the risk of dying of colorectal cancer is higher than in the general population. As compared with the general population, CD patients also die more commonly of digestive diseases in general, non-Hodgkin's lymphoma, pulmonary embolism and sepsis, and UC patients of digestive and respiratory diseases. But, for the vast, vast majority of us, IBD will not be the cause of our death.

IBD and disability

Will IBD make me disabled? A recent study from Norway showed that 19% of IBD patients were receiving a disability pension 10 years after diagnosis.[21] We measure disability taking into account such factors as quality of life and workforce participation. Compared with the general population, people with both CD and UC report poorer quality of life,[22] with the quality of life rates dropping with increased disease severity.

While the majority of people living with IBD are in the workforce, a significant percentage of us take time off work due to IBD. On average, we miss between seven and 19 days from work each year due to IBD, with more days missed in Europe than Australia.[23, 24] While from an individual's perspective this doesn't look like a lot, costs for society are large. IBD's annual cost to the European healthcare systems is estimated at €4.6-5.6 billion, and to the British healthcare system alone up to £470 million[25, 26] These costs result from the loss of productivity, absenteeism, welfare payments, early retirement, premature death and healthcare spending (e.g. hospital stays, medication). So, the answer is yes, IBD makes us disabled and this disability is costly to us personally and to the whole community in which we live. That's why it's important to seek a cure and invest in IBD research.

Key points

- IBD is a disease in which the immune system reacts in an exaggerated way to normal bacteria inhabiting the intestines, a response which may be triggered by environmental factors, or come about because someone has a genetic predisposition.
- There are three types of IBD: Crohn's disease, ulcerative colitis and indeterminate colitis. A common symptom for all three is diarrhoea but also extra-intestinal manifestations and fatigue.
- While in everyday life it may not matter much which type of IBD you have, the type of IBD may determine how well you respond to surgery.

- Over 5 million people live with IBD around the world. IBD is more common in the western and northern countries than in other parts of the world.
- It largely affects people in their twenties and is slightly more common in men than women.
- Most people living with IBD would experience at least one flare during five years of observation. In the 10 years following diagnosis, up to 50% of patients with CD will require surgery as compared with approximately 10% of those with UC.
- IBS often appears during periods of IBD remission. Psychological factors, such as anxiety, may contribute to having IBS in IBD, and counselling and psychotherapy are recommended in people having this comorbidity.
- Fatigue is very common in IBD, more so during flares than remission. Fatigue is associated with poor quality of life, anxiety and depression. Vitamin supplementation, increased physical activity, better sleep hygiene, diet and psychotherapies such as CBT are also useful.
- While the risk of colorectal cancer is increased in IBD, thanks to routine colonoscopies and good maintenance therapy the risk is decreasing.
- IBD is not a terminal illness. For both CD and UC, the risk of dying of colorectal cancer is only slightly higher than in the general population.
- IBD is more likely to lead to disability than death. Most patients work either full- or part-time, with only 20% receiving disability pension. For those who work, time off work due to IBD is at least seven days a year.

Let's now explore IBD's aetiology (causes) in a bit more depth.

Chapter 2

What causes IBD?

The role of microbiota

Chapter 1 gave a brief overview of modern theories of the causes of IBD and mentioned in particular that researchers believe that IBD happens when our bodies struggle to tolerate the bacteria inhabiting our gut. The gut is inhabited by 50–100 different types of bacteria (collectively called microbiota) totalling 100 trillion organisms. These bacteria are busy at work in the bowel; they assist digestion – aiding the absorption of nutrients and the production of vitamins – and help us deal with toxins and organisms such as yeasts (which are a type of fungus). Over thousands of years of evolution, a close and friendly relationship has developed between humans (hosts) and microbiota, in which the host dictates the activity of the bacteria and the bacteria influence the human's immunity (our defence against the organisms which are not our friends, for example viruses). This relationship is called 'mutualism' because both sides benefit.

The latest understanding of IBD is that it is caused by an incorrect reaction of our immune system to normal gut bacteria. Though these bacteria are friendly, our immune system thinks they are our enemies and thus fights them. What we also know is that the genes which predispose us to IBD are also responsible for communicating with the microbiota. Thus, IBD happens when the communication between the gut bacteria and these specific genes fails. If you sometimes argue with your partner and feel they completely miss the point, you know what I mean here. Both sides talk but the communication doesn't work.

The microbiota plays a part in ensuring that our immune system works well. For example, a bacterium called *Faecalibacterium prausnitzii* seems to have an anti-inflammatory role. When its population is reduced in the ileum (the latter part of the small intestine), this is associated with flares of CD.[1] This bacterium has shown anti-inflammatory effects in animals, and current studies are examining whether probiotics containing it are effective in managing IBD in humans. It is an attractive idea. Imagine being able to manage IBD by simply eating yoghurt! No more steroids or surgeries, just a simple diet modification. While an IBD cure is at present elusive, we are more and more certain that the gut bacteria hold the key to it.

There are two predominant views on the role of bacteria in IBD:

- that there is a disproportion between good and bad bacteria in our guts and thus treating IBD is about balancing the two
- that some bad bacteria live in the guts of those with IBD and we need to get rid of them to heal the bowel.

According to the first concept, people with IBD don't have enough bacteria such as *Faecalibacterium prausnitzii* but have too many bad bacteria, such as *Escherichia coli*. However, nothing is as simple as it initially seems, because although during flares *Faecalibacterium prausnitzii* is not particularly prevalent in some people with IBD, its reduction isn't necessary for the development of IBD. Thus, there are people who have *Faecalibacterium prausnitzii* in abundance but who still develop IBD. We also know that different gut bacteria may play a part in the course of Crohn's disease (CD), as compared with ulcerative colitis (UC), and what these bacteria do in each of the IBD sub-types may also differ.

The second concept focuses on identifying bad bacteria and specifies that there are two main culprits in IBD: MAP (*Mycobacterium avium*, subspecies *paratuberculosis*) and *Escherichia coli* (or *E coli*). Some researchers suggest that MAP causes CD. There is a cattle disease similar to IBD called Johne's disease and it is caused by MAP, so it would make sense that MAP causes IBD in humans as well. Unfortunately, when studies tried to treat IBD using an anti-MAP therapy (a sort of antibiotic) there was no improvement in IBD activity. *Escherichia coli*, on the other hand, inhabits the intestines of approximately 30% of CD sufferers and its presence is linked to flares in people after surgeries. It is, however, not an important factor in the remaining 70% of cases.

Despite this variation in results, scientists have continued to research how our microbiota could be changed for the better. There are five known ways to balance the good and the bad bacteria in our guts.

- The first one is using **pro**biotics. We could introduce the good bacteria which might fight their bad cousins and support our immune system. Products such as yoghurt, kimchi and sauerkraut include probiotics. Probiotics have been shown to be effective in ensuring that patients with UC remain in remission[2] and may thus be an interesting and low-risk treatment in UC. Unfortunately, the same cannot be said about CD, and the search for a similarly gentle treatment in CD needs to go on. In any case, at present the probiotics available on the market have low potency and thus more optimal concoctions need to be made available for the people living with UC to be able to benefit fully from this treatment.
- The second approach is using **pre**biotics, which are products that the microbiota feeds on, and thus they could

support the microbiota and benefit our digestion. Inulin and oligofructose are examples of prebiotics which support the growth of some bacteria (lactobacilli and bifidobacteria, for example), which, in turn, reduce bowel inflammation in animals.[2] Examples of foods containing prebiotics are whole grains, bananas, onions, garlic, soybeans and artichokes. We still, however, need to learn more about their role in humans before they can be considered a therapeutic option in IBD. In the meantime, there is little harm in your introducing these foods into your diet if you can tolerate them.

- The third approach is using antibiotics, which have a proven role in ensuring people with CD remain in remission, though good evidence is lacking in UC.[2] Antibiotics are not well tolerated for long periods of time (they are typically taken for 5-7 days, sometimes a few weeks), however; they may also stop working after frequent use and obviously their efficacy stops the moment you stop the treatment.

- The fourth approach is using faecal microbiota transplants (or poo transplants), which involve transplanting bacteria from healthy people to those with IBD. There is some promise to this novel technique,[3] but it is as yet uncertain which IBD patients might benefit. Again, more studies are needed.

- Finally, diet has perhaps the greatest role in ensuring we attract good bacteria.[4] Enteral nutrition (that is, the use of liquid supplements delivered by a tube directly into the stomach or small bowel) is one example of a diet change that has been well studied in IBD. It is one of the most effective treatments in paediatric CD[5] but there are not enough data to recommend it to adults and its usefulness is also questionable due to its low palatability. Imagine not being able to taste your food. Forget garlic bread, erase cheesy pizza from your memory, say goodbye to chocolate fudge. Welcome tasteless liquid delivered directly to your gut without passing through your mouth. Enteral nutrition is hardly pleasant, and so it's not difficult to see why it's not fashionable. I will discuss nutrition and diet in IBD in more detail in Chapter 11.

Gut bacteria play an important part in ensuring that our gut works well. Some of these bacteria have anti-inflammatory effects. Scientists suspect that people with IBD have too few good bacteria and too many bad ones. But simply adding good bacteria to our diet does not help all patients. In fact, probiotics have a more certain part to play in helping those living with UC than CD. As there are many species of bacteria and scientist have, to date, only glimpsed the tip of the bacterial iceberg, we don't yet know the names of all the bacteria which are beneficial for someone with IBD. Lactobacilli and bifidobacteria are currently recommended as helpful in IBD, and you can support their growth in your bowel by eating both probiotics (e.g. yoghurt) and prebiotics (fruits and vegetables such as bananas and artichokes).

I hope that by this time you can appreciate the difficulty of treating IBD. The moment one scientist comes up with an idea that works, another shows that this solution is only relevant to a small group of patients and thus cannot explain the disease fully. And thus, the search for the explanation of IBD mechanisms starts again.

The gut–brain connection

But what if the interactions between the gut bacteria and their human host are more complex than we thought? What if they also involve the brain?

We know from research on human physiology that the brain and the gut talk to each other. This communication happens via something called the brain–gut axis (or the BGA). Imagine a phone call where the radio signals are transmitted between two telephones. Similar signals are sent via our nerves, hormones and immune system between our brain and our gut.[6]

The BGA is also used by the gut bacteria to access our nervous system. According to one theory, the BGA allows our brain to decide what type of bacteria live in our guts, but at the same time our microbiota can influence the processes of our brain and, through them, our behaviour.[6] The concept that the tiny organisms that colonise our bowel can influence our mood or even personality is fascinating and is currently the subject of quite a number of studies.[7] According to these studies, stress and depression may play a part in how the microbiota communicates with our brains using the BGA. In animals, stress can influence the type of bacteria inhabiting the gut, increase inflammation and increase susceptibility to infection.[8] If stress can change the microbiota and microbiota can alter our behaviours, what if the missing link to IBD's aetiology is psychological? This is an exciting idea which I will explore further in the following chapters.

It makes sense that the brain affects what happens in our bowels and vice versa. Think of how you feel before undertaking a major journey. Rather than pleasant anticipation, even non-IBD sufferers might well feel a great deal of stress and anxiety. Will I get to the airport on time? Will there be queues to the gate? What if I can't find my passport?! It is quite common for people to report stomach aches and diarrhoea before travelling, which illustrates how our catastrophic thinking (what if I am late?) may lead to stress and that this stress contributes to digestive problems.

And what about the expression 'having butterflies in your stomach'? This feeling of fluttering in our gut is nothing else but a sign of nervousness. We know that we are stressed by having a funny feeling in one of our internal organs. However, there are also other expressions such as that something 'takes a lot of guts', meaning that we have the courage to face a dangerous situation. Having strong guts thus equals bravery. A 'gut feeling', 'go with gut', 'gut it out' – and many more similar expressions – are living proofs of the brain–gut link. But there is more to them than just folk wisdom.

Scientists have studied the brain–gut link since the nineteenth century, but particularly in the last two decades, as scientific innovations in neuroimaging have made minute observations of the brain possible. The brain communicates with the digestive tract through the autonomic nervous system, but it also links to the immune system and other systems of the body through other interconnected communication networks. This healthy communication between our brain and our gut can be disturbed through stress (and consequently anxiety and/or depression) but also through chronic inflammation.

The effect of stress, anxiety and depression on IBD

Stress, while changing how the gut behaves, can alter the way the digestive tract communicates with the brain and, subsequently, some parts of the brain become remodelled (hence, some brain structures and their functions change). What is more, communication from the gut to the brain (and specifically to the part of the brain called the 'insula' or 'insular cortex'), including the messages in relation to gut inflammation but also those messages produced by the bacteria inhabiting the gut, can affect our memory, emotions and behaviours. For example, some studies suggest that people who experience chronic intestinal inflammation are less sensitive to positive emotions – when they become sick with their IBD, their brains become rewired and they lose this sensitivity.[9] This communication system between the gut and the brain is called, as mentioned in the previous section, the BGA. Its purpose is to ensure balance within the body – in other words, to manage the external (e.g. psychological stress) and internal (e.g. gut inflammation) influences on the gastrointestinal system.

For those interested in the scientific nitty-gritty of the topic, Mayer and colleagues explain the processes behind the brain to gut signalling and the effect of chronic inflammation on both the gut and the brain in much scientific detail.[10] For anyone interested in a popular science version of the brain–gut story, Mayer recently published a fascinating book on the topic.[11]

What is stress?

As a psychologist, I have long been interested in mental health, and stress is one of the most important factors influencing it. There have been thousands of research studies conducted on stress and our understanding of it has much improved since it was first named and described by an Austrian-Canadian doctor and scientist, Hans Selye, in the 1930s.

So, what is stress? It is a feeling of being overwhelmed by a threatening event. It appears when we think we do not have the resources to cope with the event and that's why we become stressed. Stress itself doesn't have to be bad for our health. It can motivate us to come up with a solution to our problem. However, prolonged stress – where our body constantly produces hormones such as adrenaline (or epinephrine), cortisol and noradrenaline (or norepinephrine) – is not healthy and can lead to anxiety and depression, hence to potentially serious mental disorders. The 'fight or flight' response, which occurs in response to a perceived harmful event, can be recognised by a fast heartbeat, fast and shallow breathing, pupil dilation, increased sweating, tunnel vision and tense muscles, and should happen only occasionally. Yet, for many of us, because of the fast pace of life, the 'fight or flight' response is an all-day everyday occurrence. Since our bodies did not evolve to constantly tolerate the hormones released by an ongoing 'fight or flight' response, we get ill.

My first thought that stress might have something to do with the work of my digestive tract came soon after my IBD symptoms started and before I was formally diagnosed. Travel anxiety, mentioned above, had been a common occurrence in my family and thus I had some awareness of the links between stress and digestion at that basic level. When my diarrhoea had only just started, I thought that perhaps I studied too hard or had had too many exams in a short time. A few weeks later, when I lost a lot of weight, I wondered whether my parents' recent separation (amicable though it was) combined with another family event, the death of my beloved grandma, and my upcoming high school exams had anything to do with it. But after my IBD was diagnosed, I was told by my doctor that stress didn't affect my Crohn's disease, and I forgot about my gut feelings until I decided to study IBD more closely during my doctorate.

Does stress cause IBD?

What do we actually know about stress in IBD and was my doctor right in saying the two were not related?

Many studies have shown that stress has an effect on the communication between the nervous and immune systems and their connection with the gut (the BGA).[12] The vagus nerve appears to be crucial for communication between the nervous system and the gut.[8] Quite a lot of what we know of the impact of stress on bowel inflammation, and how the vagus nerve is implicated, however, comes from animal studies, as experimental studies in humans are difficult to design – people taking part in such experiments would have to be stressed for long periods of time, which is potentially dangerous and unethical. I leave you to decide whether it is ethical to stress animals, but the fact is they are the usual test subjects in medical experiments and do provide valuable insights into causation and treatment of various diseases. Thus, we cannot be certain how stress affects inflammation in humans with IBD but we have some pointers.

What we know for sure, however, is that stress is more pronounced in those who have flares of IBD than those in remission or in the healthy population. These people report that they are not only finding their IBD stressful, but they also report stressors in other areas of life (e.g. work, finances, relationships). Scientists propose that increased stress in several life areas at once may be a precursor to an IBD flare.[13] Therefore, who knows, perhaps all those negative events in my life surrounding my IBD diagnosis did play some part in its onset? But IBD is a complex disease and no single factor explains it. I now believe that these psychological stressors may have contributed to it in my case, but most likely are not its cause. My genetic predisposition, my childhood infections and repeated treatment with antibiotics, but also the urban environment I grew up in, and possibly many other factors, triggered my IBD.

On the other hand, I notice that IBD does affect mood. After years of living with it, I am tuned to my body sending me warning signs. I know that a flare is coming when my mood turns low. I am not talking here about a bad day. I mean low mood for no apparent reason for at least two weeks. In the second week, my tummy usually starts to ache, and I run to the loo more often than usual. If I increase my IBD medication at this point, I am usually able to prevent a full-blown flare. My mood returns to its healthy level a few days after my bowel movements normalise. I am not saying that that's the case for each patient. I have met quite a number of people who have told me stress was an important factor for them, but also some who didn't notice any change in their health under its influence. Again, as with nearly anything IBD-related, there is no rule for all patients. Nevertheless, for some of us, monitoring our mood can help in catching our IBD flares at the right time.

Of relevance, anxiety (with symptoms such as chronic agitation or panic attacks) and depression (low mood and inability to enjoy activities which used to give pleasure) are, in fact, very common in IBD – 19% of IBD patients report anxiety symptoms as compared with 10% of healthy controls; 21% suffer depressive symptoms versus 13% of controls.[14] However, during flares, over 60% of those living with IBD report anxiety and 35% report depressive symptoms, with those suffering CD reporting slightly higher rates than those suffering UC.

Many patients develop anxiety and depression before the onset of IBD, but a substantial proportion, particularly children, develop depression after IBD's onset.[14] Hence, it is likely that at some point in life if you have IBD you may suffer from symptoms of mental disorder.

Importantly, IBD patients who perceive their levels of stress as high often report symptoms of anxiety and depression. And, high perceived stress, anxiety and depression are associated with IBD flares and exacerbation of symptoms[15] as well as IBD hospitalisation and surgery. As such, understanding and treating mental disorders are crucial for maintaining optimal health in IBD. So, if anyone tells you stress has nothing to do with IBD, you can be sure they are not right. Stress may not cause IBD, but it may make it worse after diagnosis. Any persistent mental symptoms such as low mood, loss of interest in daily activities, anger, irritability, problems sleeping, feeling of panic and agitation, if they last for over two weeks, should not be ignored and are a reason to visit your doctor sooner rather than later.

IBD itself can be stressful; not just its diagnosis, but also its ongoing symptoms and their unpredictability, are significant stressors. Thus, the links between stress, anxiety, depression and IBD are bi-directional: IBD is associated with stress, anxiety and depression while stress, anxiety and depression may contribute to IBD's exacerbation. But there are also other factors associated with both mental health and disease activity; poor mental health often makes us change our behaviour in relation to IBD management. Those who are depressed may forget to take their IBD tablets or enemas, may miss their doctor's appointment and may neglect their diet. When depressed we simply care less about what really matters when we suffer from a chronic illness – our ongoing self-care.

Interestingly, we may be able to use these close links between our mental and physical health to our advantage. We may be able to better manage IBD's activity by treating the associated mental symptoms. The main hypothesis behind this is that, since stress is so prevalent, and many IBD patients suffer from it, if we could give people with IBD tools to cope with stress, the condition wouldn't affect them as badly as when they have limited coping strategies. Psychotherapy (talk, or talking, therapy) may be useful here as it focuses on giving people new ways to cope with life's difficulties, but antidepressants may also play a part. I discuss the role of psychotherapy and antidepressants in IBD in Chapters 9 and 12.

Key points

- Gut bacteria play an important part in ensuring that our immune system works well – that is, attacks genuine enemies and not our own cells.
- Probiotics have a clearer part to play in helping those living with UC than those with CD.
- Natural probiotics, such as fermented foods like sauerkraut, contain lactobacilli and bifidobacteria and are currently recommended as helpful in IBD, although their effects are not proven.
- The brain communicates with the gastrointestinal tract using the system called the brain–gut axis (or BGA).
- Both stress and chronic inflammation can disturb this healthy communication. What is more, communication from the gut to the brain, including the messages produced by the bacteria living in the gut, may influence our emotions, and often not for the better.
- Stress is a feeling of being overwhelmed by a threatening event.
- Stress is more pronounced in those who have flares in their IBD than those in remission or in healthy people.
- Increased stress may be a precursor to an IBD flare, but also to anxiety and depression.
- The relationship between stress and IBD is bi-directional – stress is associated with flares and having IBD can cause stress.
- Any mental symptoms, such as low mood, loss of interest in daily activities, anger, irritability, problems sleeping, feelings of panic and agitation, if they last for over two weeks, should not be ignored and are a reason to visit your doctor.

Part II

Living with IBD

Chapter 3

The psychological impact of IBD

Diagnosis of IBD and its ongoing symptoms have an impact on practically every aspect of life. Psychological research quite often uses the composite term 'quality of life' in order to be able to describe disease burden and compare it between different illnesses. As I have discussed in Chapter 2, IBD is well known to negatively affect quality of life.[1] IBD's incurability and unpredictability, disease activity, medication side-effects, hospitalisations and associated surgery are the obvious culprits, but there are also other factors explaining low quality of life in IBD: poor mental health, negative self-image and sexuality, coping difficulties, poor social functioning and stigma.[1]

In one of my latest studies,[2] common patient concerns included: isolation, threat to general lifestyle, uncertain future, pain, constant use of medicines, cancer, possibility of surgery, body image, fear of flare, incontinence, lack of control, impact on family, career and social life, travelling, diet, mortality, and others. These are all valid concerns and many of them are discussed in this book. Hopefully, by increasing your understanding of IBD, they will not be as troubling to you in the future.

I addressed mental health in Chapter 2 and will only add now that those IBD patients who report significant stress, and those with anxiety and depression as well as those with active disease, report poorer quality of life than IBD patients without these problems or the healthy population.[3] Self-image and sexuality are important topics in their own right and are discussed in detail in Chapter 5.

Coping strategies

How do you cope? Coping with IBD relates to our ability to manage its demands and these can be complex – physical (e.g. symptoms), psychological (e.g. anxiety), social (e.g. our ability to work). We all use a variety of coping strategies in daily life and if this topic interests you, read any textbook of health psychology[4] to learn about how much research has been done on coping in general and with health problems. Coping helps us to reduce the burden of a chronic illness, such as IBD.

- If we successfully reduce the burden of IBD and worry about it less, we call it 'adaptive' coping.
- If, however, our coping mechanisms are not useful, and they don't reduce the stress of IBD, or reduce it at a great cost such as addiction, they are called 'maladaptive' and these are particularly dangerous to anyone suffering from a chronic illness.

Of relevance to IBD, we know that if someone with the condition uses emotion-focused coping (explained below) this has worse psychological outcomes than using problem-focused coping.[5]

- Emotion-focused coping is about reducing the distress caused by a situation in which we find ourselves (e.g. dealing with an IBD flare). We can say that we use emotion-focused coping if we avoid thinking about IBD, deny the existence of its symptoms, or when we distract ourselves from thinking about IBD by using alcohol or recreational drugs.
- Problem-focused coping, on the other hand, attempts to

deal with the source of our stress, when we confront the problem or seek further information. Ideally, problem-focused coping aims to remove the cause of the stress.

I want to highlight that emotion-focused coping is not universally bad for us and problem-focused coping is not always helpful. For example, when you have to go through a painful procedure, it is very healthy to use distraction. Medical hypnosis, meditation and relaxation are common types of emotion-focused techniques to help deal with unpleasant sensations. When you focus your attention on something other than pain, the pain becomes less severe. Denying that you suffer from IBD and pretending you don't need to take your medications, however, wouldn't help you and would thus be considered maladaptive coping. If you deny IBD's existence or refuse treatment, you will only become more ill.

In contrast, problem-focused coping may not always be practical. For example, there is no known way to cure IBD, so you cannot remove your main stressor. You can learn more about it, however, which – as you may recall – is my method of coping with IBD. That's why I study and write about it. I confront it daily, monitor my symptoms, take my medications, undergo colonoscopy when it's required and, altogether, accept that I have it. But when the doctor's examination hurts me I focus on my breathing or talk to the doctor to distract myself. Does that make sense?

IBD and social life

Social support is another important psychological dimension. In general, IBD patients feel they are well supported by their families and friends and their level of support is greater than that of the general population. Social support is now the topic of many research studies as it seems that lack of it may be comparable to smoking in terms of its impact on health. Numerous studies have shown that loneliness substantially increases our chances of dying and that it can be as harmful to our health as cigarettes![6] IBD-specific research shows that high levels of social support improve the clinical course of CD.[7] It is an interesting finding because it is modifiable. If we feel lonely, we can do something about it. We can reach out to other people, either through our family connections or by meeting new people through a variety of activities – sport, learning a new language, cooking, art classes, book clubs – and we could do it even when we have limited financial resources, as local councils and public libraries have low- or no-cost offerings. The internet is one cheap source of contacts – most libraries now offer access to it free of charge – and while it has not been studied extensively in IBD, research to date demonstrates a beneficial role for online support groups for IBD patients.[8]

Despite the high level of social support that people living with IBD receive, we frequently report social functioning as challenging. And no wonder! Our preoccupation with toilets must appear bizarre to new acquaintances. Stigma associated with IBD may prevent us from revealing our diagnosis to people around us. Diarrhoea, bloating and gas are not commonplace topics which one mentions in a random conversation with strangers, or in a tearoom at work. We don't even discuss them that often with people close to us – bowel functions are a taboo subject in many cultures.

For me personally, as I have lived with IBD and worked in this area for many years, the taboo is long gone. I was reminded recently about it when I was picking up my husband and his colleague from the train station after some work event. The colleague asked me out of courtesy how I was doing and, as I wasn't doing particularly well at the time, I started describing my stomach problems without much thought. The poor man paled and then blushed and turned mute. I stopped when I saw my husband hiding a smile. He later told me: 'Too much detail, darling.' We both laughed for quite some time recalling the discomfort I quite innocently created for this colleague. As a rule, I do admit publicly I have IBD, but I do know now that I shouldn't always describe how it affects me. Some people are not ready for it!

Social gatherings are another source of social problems. Many family events, such as birthdays or weddings, revolve around food. And people living with IBD frequently adopt a particular diet. Some can't tolerate lactose and thus avoid dairy; others can't digest some types of meat; yet others may not tolerate specific foods like onion, mushrooms or chocolate. (I discuss diet in IBD in Chapter 11.) We may not want to tell everyone about IBD, and so misunderstandings may arise when we refuse to eat what we are served. Some of us never go to restaurants, dreading asking a thousand questions: is the waiter quite certain garlic is not part of the signature dish or is the mayonnaise dressing in my Caesar salad definitely lactose-free?

On a practical note, one of the other things that is always on an IBD sufferer's mind is proximity and ease of access to toilets. When I travel to a new place for work, my level of stress is always heightened until I learn my way around the local loos. During holidays, when I am in tourist spots where there may be queues for restrooms, I do use toilet locator apps (see the Self-help resource section on page 134 for details). Travel loses some of its spontaneity, but at least you get peace of mind.

IBD and employment

Patients often ask me if it's wise to make your IBD known at work. Patient organisations, such as Crohn's & Colitis Australia and Crohn's & Colitis UK, offer booklets dedicated to the issue, so I won't spend a lot of time on it. Not every work environment is supportive, not every boss understanding, but it does make your life easier when you don't have to hide IBD. I go a step further, as not only do my colleagues know about my IBD, but I frequently tell my students.

There are two reasons for doing so – the first is so that they can see that a person with a chronic illness can have a successful career; the second is more practical: I may need to break the lecture to run to the loo and want to reassure them that that's normal. I usually ask new student cohorts how they would respond if their teacher excused herself for five minutes to go to the loo. I do it to verify my belief that there is no need to fear going to the loo even when you have a work meeting or a lecture. Most people don't mind. Yet, most of my patients fear it and some would rather miss university or work when there is a chance they might need a toilet break.

My students, year after year, tell me it is fine. They can take care of themselves for five minutes. Of course, I do teach adults and IBD may be more problematic to those who teach in primary schools, but there are ways to help yourself if you share your IBD diagnosis with at least one of your colleagues who can replace you in case of an emergency. Thus, my advice would be to share your IBD at least with one person you can count on at work and ideally share it with your boss – the latter will save you explaining your sick days or meeting interruptions (if you or the boss are concerned about them).

Diet is another complication in the work environment – think of those of us who are required to have regular lunches with clients. If you know the restaurant where you are going, you can check the menu by calling the venue beforehand, but what if your client likes hot Indian food?

A few years ago, I was an invited speaker at a meeting in London and my British colleagues wanted to thank me for coming by inviting me to a traditional Bangladeshi restaurant. They were particularly keen on it as it was considered one of the best in town. I felt anxious just by scanning the menu on the internet. Curry, unless prepared by myself, is usually a no-no and you don't want to go through three days of upset stomach during an overseas trip. I wondered what to do. In the end I did thank them for coming up with a great idea but suggested an Italian or Greek place instead. I did reveal I had IBD to my host and we ended up in a Greek taverna which offered one of the best grilled octopus I have ever had. So, it paid off to be assertive.

But IBD does have an impact on work, study and pleasure beyond our choices of food. Our symptoms may be severe. We may be sick or simply exhausted and so unable to engage in everyday functioning. Despite these objective difficulties, however, those with IBD are as likely to be employed as those in the community (though admittedly they miss more days of work).

Personality and IBD

To close on the topic of IBD's psychological impact, I think I should mention personality. It is not a big topic in IBD research but there have been a few studies examining it.[9] A personality trait of neuroticism (a tendency to interpret situations as threatening – in the context of IBD you may, for example, take every bout of diarrhoea as a certain sign of an upcoming flare and worry about it a lot) has been linked to reduced quality of life, and worse emotional and social functioning in IBD. There have also been some studies into a personality factor called alexithymia (inability to identify and describe emotions of our own and others) which has been linked to poor adjustment to having IBD. If you have high neuroticism or are alexithymic, you may take longer to adjust to IBD and may need to work harder to strengthen your coping mechanisms, but having these traits does not predict your IBD outcomes in any other way, so don't worry if you are a worrier or struggle to describe what you feel.

Key points

- IBD is well known to negatively affect quality of life. IBD patients who report significant stress, those with anxiety and depression, and those with active disease report poorer quality of life than IBD patients without these problems or the healthy population.
- Coping with IBD is all about our ability to manage its demands. A type of coping when we avoid thinking about IBD, deny the existence of its symptoms, or distract ourselves from thinking about it by using alcohol or recreational drugs is called 'maladaptive coping'. Improving knowledge of IBD is an example of useful or 'adaptive' coping.
- Social support is important for both our mental and physical health. Strong social support networks have been shown to improve the clinical course of IBD, so being social helps your bowel. Being open about having IBD often helps negotiate social situations and can be useful in the work environment.

Chapter 4

IBD in children and adolescents

It was shortly before my seventeenth birthday when I suddenly started losing weight. I had always loved food and my appetite didn't change; if anything, I felt hungrier than ever. I did as much sport as always, swimming a few times a week and playing tennis, but my weight dropped. I also had diarrhoea, which my parents initially attributed to a stomach bug. After six or seven weeks of these symptoms my aunt, our family doctor, started worrying and she referred me for a blood test. Its result was alarming. My inflammation marker was exceedingly high; my haemoglobin and my iron levels were very low (see Self-help resources on page 131 for information on how to interpret blood tests). Within a couple of weeks, I ended up in hospital. I was given a drug called sulphasalazine (see Chapter 9). After the first few doses, my body became covered with red, measles-like pimples and the doctors concluded I was allergic to it. There was no alternative available, however, as at that time 5ASA drugs, such as mesalazine, were not funded by the Polish healthcare system.

Mesalazine was impossible to buy locally and so my archaeologist father sought help from his colleagues based in Germany, who helped us buy the drug there and import it to Poland. While waiting for the delivery of this medication, I was drugged with some strong antihistamines and mostly slept for two weeks.

I took these mesalazine tablets and suppositories for several months and tolerated them well, but they cost my parents a fortune. Poland was still a poor post-communist country and the financial burden of importing these medications from Germany every month was not insignificant. My parents both worked in the public sector. Luckily, at some point we discovered there was an American pharmacy in Warsaw which sold mesalazine, the cost of which was not as high as buying it in Germany.

Months passed but my IBD was not completely controlled. Steroids were the next suggestion, but my parents saw them as a last resort. They wanted to avoid giving me drugs which had several pages' worth of side effects (see Chapter 9). I was still developing. My parents dreaded the impact on my bones and the increased risk of infections. As I was in love for the first time, my only worry was weight gain and moon face – when your face becomes round, full or puffy. I pictured myself becoming a strongman with no neck and that, I concluded, was not an option. I preferred to suffer tummy aches indefinitely, but luckily my parents had more sense and could see further than the possibility of their daughter becoming less beautiful for a few months. They explored other options.

A doctor suggested changing my environment. Poland has a temperate climate, with long, cold and gloomy winters. I think the doctor's hypothesis must have been that my low vitamin D levels contributed to poor IBD outcomes. Fortunately, my father's specialty was the Mediterranean. We spent a few weeks in Tunisia, and the sun, rest and a different diet did make some difference to my health. I was still incredibly thin – when one of my cousins saw me in a bathing suit she started crying and told me I looked as if I was about to disappear. But in Tunisia I gained enough energy to let me take my final high school exam and pass the university entry tests back in Poland.

Unfortunately, the stress must have been too great – I was always over-ambitious and wouldn't be happy merely passing the exams. My IBD flared soon afterwards and no amount of mesalazine could help.

My father then contacted a friend in the UK and sought medical advice on my treatment there. He was ready to take me to Britain to search for a cure, but a wise British doctor said he did not recommend it. He advised that steroids were the best option, and these could be obtained cheaply in Poland, with no need to spend a fortune seeking private treatment overseas. This would have meant my parents taking out a loan, so I was relieved that the doctor had some sense and was not greedy. I was already 19 by then. Growth retardation was no longer a fear. It was summer, so not a 'flu season, and since I didn't have to be much in public due to vacations, how I looked was not important. The timing was perfect.

I took steroids for three months. They were a miracle treatment. I got my energy back. My diarrhoea disappeared. My iron and haemoglobin returned to normal. I became moody though, and, as I had predicted, my face became huge. It didn't help that the nasty piece of work, my boyfriend, left me just when my IBD was getting worse. But I had lovely friends and family around me and altogether I don't have bad memories of my first steroid treatment. It helped me lead a normal life for three years afterwards.

What I wanted to demonstrate with my personal story is that IBD impacts hugely on the family of a child with IBD. Parents are desperate to find a cure and will pay any price for a promise of improvement. As I was in my teens when IBD started, at least I could have been trusted to take myself to a doctor and remember to take my medication. The burden of IBD on the family of a small child who requires their parents' care with even the simplest tasks is hard to describe. Through my research and psychological work, I have spoken to many parents of children suffering from IBD. Their helplessness and grief at witnessing their child suffering are heart-wrenching each time.

The outlook for children and adolescents with IBD

What I tell the parents I meet, as a way of reassurance, is that while there is no cure as yet for IBD, the treatment is getting better. Trust me, it is easier to have a child with IBD now than it was 20 or 30 years ago, when the only options were steroids, sulphasalazine and/or surgery. In time, as the child and their family learn how to manage IBD and spot the early warning signs of a flare, and as they accept the psychological ups and downs of the illness, it is never as bad as during the initial phase of the disease. IBD becomes a part of life and this life doesn't have to be worse or less meaningful than if the child was completely healthy.

For most patients, there are periods of remission, sometimes for several years. In these times, we are free of symptoms and we only differ from our peers in that we take some maintenance medication. Children with IBD grow up, finish schools, get jobs, travel, and start families of their own. By observing the famous people living with IBD, such as singer Anastacia, or five-time gold medal Olympic Champion Sir Steve Redgrave, or Australian champion surfer Brittani Nichols, we can learn that IBD does not prevent you from being successful. As with any life experience, it will only be whatever you make of it. So, if you are a parent of an IBD child, don't despair. Remember that there are good resources available and these can guide you in how to help your child (see Self-help resources on page 133).

Better resources are becoming available because IBD in children is becoming a public concern, as some 25% of new IBD cases are in children under the age of 18 years and the incidence of paediatric IBD is on the rise.[1] Crohn's disease (CD) is more common in children than ulcerative colitis (UC).

Unfortunately, IBD presenting in early age is typically more severe and extensive than in adults. It may interfere with growth, psychosocial and sexual development, and education. Up to 40% of children with the condition experience growth failure, which results from poor nutrition, problems absorbing nutrients, chronic inflammation and treatment with corticosteroids. As doctors are well aware of the risk of growth failure, in the first instance a child diagnosed with CD is typically started on an exclusively liquid diet, which usually has good effects,[2] but in adolescents with extensive disease a more complex therapy is typically prescribed (e.g. biologics – see Chapter 9). Some of these treatments given in adolescence may influence fertility in the future and thus their long-term impact needs to be discussed at the outset of therapy.

The impact on mental health

IBD at any stage of life requires adjustment, but the impact on psychosocial development is unique in young people. Children with IBD (similarly to children with other chronic illnesses) report more behavioural and emotional problems than their healthy counterparts. A significant number of children present with mental illnesses, such as depression, in addition to their IBD (10–23%), and many have poorer quality of life than their healthy peers.[3] In young people with IBD, poorer quality of life is often found to be related to embarrassment resulting from frequent use of toilets and becoming a target of 'bathroom humour' by their peer group. Looking at the coping strategies employed by kids and adolescents with IBD, there are very few studies which explore this issue, and what we know is only that young people with IBD appear to have less well-developed coping skills than their healthy counterparts.

Social functioning is another important issue in young people suffering from IBD. In the eyes of their parents, adolescents with IBD have similar social lives to their healthy peers but when we ask the young people themselves, they report the opposite – that their social life is not that great. Reassuringly, however, studies examining self-esteem in young people with IBD showed no difference in its levels between IBD patients, healthy controls and young people with other chronic conditions.[4]

Key points

- At present, 25% of new IBD cases are in young people under the age of 18 years, with CD more prevalent in this group than UC.
- A large proportion of children living with IBD experience growth failure, a consequence of poor nutrition, problems with absorbing nutrients, chronic inflammation and treatment with corticosteroids.
- Children with IBD report more behavioural and emotional problems than their healthy counterparts, with many suffering from depression. Parents should not hesitate to seek psychological support when needed.
- Remember, emotional difficulties are as much a symptom of IBD as diarrhoea and do not reflect badly on you or your child.

Chapter 5

Sexuality, fertility and pregnancy in IBD

While the incidence of IBD in children is rising, IBD is most common in adults, and particularly people in their twenties or thirties. What could be a more adult-specific topic than sex?

Sexuality

IBD does affect our sexuality and not for the better. Up to 75% of women and 44% of men report sexual dysfunction due to IBD. In consequence, the frequency of sexual activity is decreased in IBD patients, with more women reporting a negative impact.

Why are sexual problems common in people living with IBD? It starts with our negative body image – visible disease (e.g. anal fistulas), steroids making us fat, stomas (i.e. an opening in your tummy which diverts your faeces into a bag), and extra-intestinal manifestations (inflammation of skin, for example) contribute to our dissatisfaction with our bodies. As sexuality has much to do with sexual attraction, these changes to our bodies undermine our self-confidence. It's therefore not surprising that as many as 60% of IBD patients, particularly women who have undergone surgery, report impaired body image.

Many women report IBD's negative impact on their partner relationships[1] and sexual problems play a part here. Libido is reduced in patients with IBD, most commonly in women, those after surgery, and those with active disease. However, some recent research shows that sexuality may improve in many people post-surgery,[2] so don't avoid surgery on account of possible sexual problems. The most important factor influencing sexuality in IBD is, in fact, coexisting depression.[3] Depressed women with IBD report lower libido, diminished orgasm and reduced frequency of intercourse. This link between psychology and sexuality is important, as depression can be successfully treated, improving sexuality in turn.

In men with IBD who report sexual problems, erectile dysfunction is associated with disease activity.[4] In women, dyspareunia (i.e. painful sexual intercourse) is common,[5] particularly when IBD is confined to the anal area. Some of the sexual problems may be attributed to the IBD medication – methotrexate has been associated with impotence, steroids with sexual dysfunctions in women and biological agents (i.e. anti-TNF alpha) with sexual dysfunction in men (see Chapter 9). However, IBD medications are not generally known to have a large effect on sexuality, and so the biggest culprits are our blue mood and negative self-perception.

It is crucial in this context that IBD patients communicate with their partners about their sexual difficulties and that both parties can voice their concerns and questions openly – as an IBD patient, do not assume it is only you who are terrified and embarrassed. Your partner may struggle as well – they do love you and so don't want to hurt you. Reach out to them and do not fear discussing your concerns. If you and your partner struggle with sex, consider seeing a counsellor, or if IBD seems to be at the core of the issue (as is often the case soon after having stoma surgery) speak to your IBD nurse, your stoma nurse or your IBD doctor.

Contraception

As planned conception is best in IBD (to avoid conceiving during flares), contraception is important and over 80% of IBD patients use some form of it. However, very few IBD patients discuss their family planning with their IBD specialists, but this should happen early in treatment. There is no research that I am aware of on contraception in men with IBD, but here is what we know about it in women.

There is good evidence that in healthy people, use of the oral contraceptive pill increases the risk of developing IBD.[6] However, if one already suffers from IBD, does taking the pill make it worse? According to a recent systematic review, there is no increase in flare frequency or severity in women taking the pill,[7] but very few studies have been conducted in the area so watch this space as the conclusion may change.

What about the risk of venous thromboembolism (VTE, the formation of blood clots in a vein)? The risk of this condition is increased in IBD in general[8] and oral contraceptive pills that include the hormone oestrogen are known to increase it further. The data at present are not very comprehensive and the recommendation is that if you have planned surgery scheduled you should cease taking the pill four weeks prior to the operation. When surgery is not planned, the pill can be taken by women with mild IBD only. In those with active or extensive IBD, those taking steroids, those who are immobilised, and those with vitamin deficiencies, an alternative method of contraception is recommended. Alternatives include progesterone-only pills, implants, and injectable or intrauterine contraceptives, as these are not associated with an increased risk of VTE.[9]

Since women with IBD often have diarrhoea, is the pill a reliable method of contraception? If your disease is active, you may need to use alternatives to the pill, such as implants. The general advice for women using oral contraceptives, who have been vomiting or have had severe diarrhoea for more than 24 hours, is to assume the effectiveness of the pill has been compromised and to follow instructions for missed pills.

What about other methods of contraception? Barrier methods, such as condoms, have similar efficacy as in the healthy population, but they are less fool-proof than hormonal contraception and thus may not be appropriate when teratogenic (potentially causing birth defects) IBD medication, such as methotrexate, is used. Laparoscopic sterilisation is not a good option in IBD if you have had previous IBD-related surgery as there may be complications.[10] Intrauterine devices appear generally safe.[11]

We know what to do if we don't want to have a baby, but what if we do?

Fertility

The common factors which limit fertility (i.e. our ability to produce offspring) in IBD are abstinence or reduced sexual activity due to pain, fear of incontinence or body image. But when we overcome these, and as long as we are in remission, we are as likely to conceive as healthy people. If, however, our IBD (particularly CD) is flaring when we try to conceive, our fertility will be reduced.[12]

Nevertheless, IBD patients have fewer children than their healthy counterparts. This is due to voluntary childlessness, often dictated by fear of passing IBD on to the child, concerns regarding the effect of IBD drugs on the foetus and the fear of congenital abnormalities.

If a woman decides she wants to get pregnant, she often stops her IBD treatment, which in turn may lead to a flare. Stopping your treatment and thus inviting a flare is not a good idea because flares may negatively impact the outcome for the child. Thus, all efforts need to be made to continue with IBD treatment. Discuss your treatment and your concerns with your doctor, change to a safer alternative if needed, but don't go cold turkey!

Another factor that can affect fertility is IBD surgery, with female UC patients having much lower fertility after some types of surgery.[13] For example, infertility rates increase from 20% to 63% after ileal pouch-anal anastomosis (IPAA), as some women develop what are called 'adhesions' which disturb the function of the fallopian tubes. If you plan to have children and are about to have a surgery, discuss the risks with your doctor.

For males, there is no increased risk of infertility, though after ileal pouch-anal surgery some erectile and ejaculation problems may occur.[2] Largely, however, IBD has no impact on male sexual function. The only factor that is important in terms of male fertility is medication (see below, specifically sulphasalazine and methotrexate).

Conception and pregnancy

As many patients are diagnosed with IBD in their twenties and thirties, pregnancy is a relatively common occurrence in those living with IBD. For the majority of sufferers, pregnancy will go well but it's important to understand what impact IBD may have on the baby and its health.

Typically, when we decide we want to have a baby, our gastroenterologist should discuss risky behaviours (drinking, smoking and drugs). This is relevant to any pregnancy and not just to IBD patients, of course, but healthy women won't be talking to a gastroenterologist. Then, your nutrition should be discussed as your IBD may mean you don't absorb certain vitamins and other nutrients, such as folic acid (vitamin B9), iron or vitamin B12. Your fertility will also be discussed in the context of your disease activity and medication. Heredity, a genetic risk of passing IBD to your children, should also be talked about, as many people worry about it. This risk is not high, but it does exist. In children with one parent affected by IBD, the risk is no greater than 7%[14] while in the case of both parents with IBD, it is up to 36%.[15] Then, mode of delivery and breastfeeding should also be addressed. When you are pregnant, a follow-up with your doctor is recommended every two months if you remain in remission. If you flare, the follow-up should occur every two weeks. You will have blood tests and endoscopy if necessary. If you cannot conceive in 12 months, you are usually referred to a fertility clinic.

The impact of pregnancy on IBD

If you become pregnant during remission, your risk of flare is the same as in non-pregnant IBD women (so approximately 30% of women will flare). If, however, this is not the case and you become pregnant during a flare, you are at a high risk of persistent IBD activity throughout your pregnancy. Thus, pregnancy may influence the course of your IBD.[16]

While pregnancy presents risks in women with active IBD, it may also have positive effects on the long-term course of your IBD. The more children we have, the lower the need for surgery and resections in IBD.[16] Some studies report that mothers with CD flare less often after pregnancy than before. So that's some encouraging news.

Medication during conception and pregnancy

IBD medication is a typical concern around pregnancy. Women generally want to take as few medications as possible but uncontrolled IBD is more harmful to the baby than most of the commonly used IBD treatments. Active IBD may negatively affect placenta development and lead to preterm birth and low birth weight. Here is what we know about IBD treatment and pregnancy.

- Generally, the majority of IBD treatments taken during pregnancy and lactation are associated with low risk of complications for the baby.
- 5ASA drugs (see Chapter 9) are safe in pregnancy and there is no need to stop them. If you are a woman taking sulphasalazine during pregnancy, you may need to take folic acid as well. In males, sulphasalazine influences the quality of sperm and should be replaced with another 5ASA for the period of conception.
- Thiopurines (e.g. azathioprine) are most likely safe in males and females, with no increased risk of malformations;[17] however, an increased risk of preterm birth has been noted. Despite this, patients are advised to continue their thiopurine treatment during pregnancy as the risks are low.
- Methotrexate use by pregnant women has been associated with congenital malformations.[18] However, if you become pregnant while taking it, the options should be discussed with the doctor prescribing it. In men, there is a limited risk of producing offspring with major congenital malformations,[19] but methotrexate does negatively affect fertility and is not recommended three to six months before conception so you will want to find an alternative as soon as you know you want to try for a baby.
- While there have been very few IBD-related studies, cyclosporine during pregnancy is not associated with congenital malformations.[16]
- If your IBD flares during pregnancy, steroids are typically given, with enemas, foams and suppositories being safer means of drug delivery for the baby than oral steroids. In the first trimester, the use of steroids has been associated with some malformations in newborns.[20] In late pregnancy, there is a chance that the newborn will stop producing their own corticosteroids and they should be checked for this after birth. Nevertheless, some steroids are safer than

others, with prednisolone being generally regarded as safe
during pregnancy.

- Anti-TNF alpha agents are not associated with an
  increased risk of congenital malformations. Infliximab and
  adalimumab (also known as biologics) are both safe in the
  short term, but long-term risks for the developing immune
  system and for infections in children are as yet unknown.
  However, as these drugs cross the placenta, if a woman is
  in remission, she may be advised to stop taking anti-TNF
  alpha drugs around gestational week 22.
- Antibiotics such as metronidazole and ciprofloxacin, while
  generally safe, should be avoided in the first trimester due
  to a slightly increased risk of congenital abnormalities.[16]
- Anti-diarrhoeal agents, such as loperamide, should be used
  with caution, particularly late in pregnancy as the newborn
  may experience withdrawal symptoms.
- Bile-salt binders, vitamins and minerals are largely safe
  during pregnancy.

Mode of delivery

While women with IBD are 1.5 times more likely to undergo
caesarean section[21] than their healthy counterparts, most women
with IBD experience normal pregnancies, with vaginal delivery
considered the safest option. The exceptions to this rule are
women who have had an ileostomy (a type of surgical removal
of part of the ileum, the final part of the small intestine) and
those whose IBD is confined to the perianal area and rectum,
particularly if fistulas are present. In these women, a caesarean
section may be a safer option.

Whether a child is delivered vaginally or through a caesarean
section, its risk of inheriting IBD is the same. However, we now
know that caesarean section may affect the child's immunity.
During a natural delivery, the baby is exposed to its mother's

vaginal and faecal bacteria. These bacteria become part of the baby's microbiota (including its gut bacteria). During a caesarean section, where the baby does not pass through the birth canal, such exposure to the mother's bacteria is not possible. There are some studies showing the benefits of giving a baby born by caesarean a swab of vaginal fluid to support the building of their microflora, but this practice is not yet part of routine care post-caesarean delivery as more research is needed. Watch this space.

Outcomes of pregnancy

While the majority of pregnancies have good outcomes, for women with IBD there is an increased risk of premature delivery. Low birth weight (<2500 g) is twice as likely in the offspring of women suffering from IBD as in those of healthy women,[21] and the risk of congenital abnormalities is also slightly increased. Disease activity at conception and during pregnancy is an important risk factor for negative pregnancy outcomes and that's why women with IBD should plan their pregnancies according to disease activity.

Key points

- Most women and nearly half of men report sexual dysfunction due to IBD. Impaired body image is common as is lower libido. The latter is often a sign of depression and psychological support can help here. Open communication between partners around IBD's effects on sexuality may also help.
- While the majority of IBD patients use contraception, very few discuss family planning with their IBD specialists. Given that diarrhoea is common in IBD, the pill is not always the most effective contraceptive method, and implants or intrauterine devices may be a better option.
- IBD patients in remission have similar fertility rates to healthy people.
- When a woman with IBD gets pregnant, she should not stop IBD treatment. Most types of IBD treatments are safe in pregnancy and going cold turkey may do more harm than good.
- Pregnancies in women with IBD usually end well, with women largely having a natural birth (the exception are women who have undergone ileostomy and those with IBD in the perianal area and rectum – caesarean section is the preferred option here).
- A precondition for good outcomes in pregnancy is conception during remission. Pregnancy has positive effects on the long-term course of IBD. The more children we have, the lower the need for surgery and resections.
- The risk of passing your IBD to a child is small when one parent only has the condition, and increases to 36% with both parents affected by IBD.

Chapter 6

IBD in the over 60s

Up to 30% of new IBD cases are among those aged over 60,[1] yet IBD's diagnosis may be delayed in older populations as it is considered a disease of the young. Consequently, patients may go untreated for a period of time, which poses its own risks. While those who were diagnosed when they were younger continue to manage their IBD through their later years using the coping strategies they have already developed, new patients may find IBD hard to deal with in later life. Research in this population is quite limited, and thus the recommendations for overall management of the condition are often borrowed from other chronic illnesses more common in older age than IBD.

Problems specific to older patients with IBD

A range of problems related to increasing age may complicate IBD in the over sixties:

- Diarrhoea followed by malnutrition and dehydration, as well as pain, add to fatigue which is a common problem with increasing age.
- Other chronic conditions which the patient may suffer from in addition to IBD may complicate IBD's treatment – for example, though it is uncommon, IBD medications may interact with medications for another illness. In addition,

some treatments need to be avoided – for example, commonly used over-the-counter painkillers are linked to IBD flares[2] and their use needs to be limited.

- Administration of IBD medication (by injection or enemas, for example) may be difficult due to physical impairment.
- Running to the toilet to avoid IBD accidents may end in a fall and fractured bones; thus IBD may cause an accident of a different and usually more serious nature.
- If still in the workforce, job security may be threatened due to IBD as those only recently diagnosed with the condition may need frequent doctor's appointments and sick leave.
- Older patients who live alone are known to have worse health outcomes than those sharing a home with someone, and social isolation, the risk of which increases with age, can be a barrier to treatment.
- Older patients may not be able to get to the doctor easily without help and thus may not see their doctor as often as they feel is needed.
- They may also forget about their treatment and become non-adherent – dementia is increasingly common in the general population as we now live longer, and it may complicate IBD.

In some communities, where IBD is stigmatised, older IBD patients may not like to admit they suffer from it and thus avoid exposure through limiting contacts with healthcare professionals. On the other hand, if willing to seek medical help, a potential barrier to treatment is the age difference between the patient and their often much younger doctor. Of relevance here is what I discuss in Chapter 7 about the patient–doctor relationship: this relationship may suffer if the doctor has little experience of working with older patients or dedicates too little time to their visits. If the doctor–patient relationship doesn't work, it's best to find another health practitioner. However, I admit this is potentially more problematic in this patient group, as some older people may be limited to their local practice due to lack of support in travelling further afield.

Depending on the country, medication may need to be purchased and this poses a significant burden, particularly on those who have already retired and with limited financial resources. Some IBD treatments, such as biologics, are very pricey and unaffordable unless covered by the healthcare system.

How should older IBD patients be treated?

Unlike younger patients, the main goal of treatment for older patients is symptom control as opposed to healing inflammation. Complete healing of inflammation may only be achieved using very aggressive treatments which can pose significant risks in older patients.[3] Thus, a conservative approach is usually applied, where good quality of life is a more important therapeutic goal than low levels of inflammation.

In terms of general support for dealing with the diagnosis of IBD and coping with the disease on a daily basis, psychologists and other mental health professionals can be of huge help and can make the transition to living with IBD smoother. Some IBD clinics offer such services or you can be referred by your GP. I discuss particular psychotherapeutic approaches in Chapter 12.

Many general medical clinics now offer appointments with geriatricians, the doctors who specialise in helping the older population, and their services could be used if there are problems in communication with other health professionals or if you simply want a bit more time with the doctor.

Key points

- Up to 30% of new IBD cases are among those aged over 60.
- Other chronic conditions that the patient may suffer from in addition to IBD, such as dementia, may complicate IBD treatment.
- IBD medications may interact with medications for another illness and some treatments need to be avoided – for example, regular use of over-the-counter painkillers is not advised in IBD treatment for older people as it may lead to flares.
- Good quality of life and thus symptom control is a more important therapeutic goal in older patients with IBD than low levels of inflammation.
- Social isolation may be a barrier to treatment in IBD as may an age difference between the patient and a much younger doctor. It's best to choose a geriatrician or a doctor who has experience working with the older population.
- If you struggle adjusting to IBD, do not hesitate to ask for support such as from psychologists, social workers or counsellors, either in person or over the phone.

Part III

Treating IBD

Chapter 7

Healthcare models for IBD

Different cultural responses to health

IBD affects people in all corners of the Earth. It can be more or less common, as explained in Chapter 1, but there is no country or culture where IBD does not exist.

When I moved to South Australia from Poland it quickly became clear to me that health matters were more of a taboo there than in the part of the world where I was raised. Polish people are obsessed with health and discuss it frequently and, by and large, openly – the exception is serious mental illness, such as schizophrenia, but depression or anxiety are very much in the open, particularly in big cities, where undergoing psychotherapy is quite fashionable. I think there are more pharmacies than patisseries in Poland and, believe me, the latter are omnipresent as the nation boasts a sweet tooth like none other.

South Australians, in my experience, are more private about their health. They share their concerns only after getting to know you well, and many health problems, such as depression, but also gastrointestinal conditions, are still considered stigmatising. On the other hand, drug use is more widely accepted in Australia even by the older generation, whereas my parents' generation in Poland (those born in the 1950s) fear recreational drugs. That's one reason why Polish people get suspicious when it comes to legalising medical marijuana; they were taught all drugs were evil and so they express major concerns regarding legalising marijuana, no matter how effective it might be for cancer-related pain.

These, of course, are my personal, and possibly biased observations, but culture does determine our beliefs and decisions in relation to health.[1] Our relationship with health practitioners, attitudes towards therapy and also our perceptions of sensations such as pain are also influenced by it.[2]

Early in my academic career I conducted neuropsychological research on trauma and worked with a clinician from former Yugoslavia. Like me, she was an immigrant in Australia, and she shared with me some cross-cultural observations regarding pain perceptions in her patients. To her surprise, she had observed that Australians reported less pain than the patients she treated who had emigrated from Eastern Europe. Not only did Aussies complain less about trauma-related pain; they seemed not to feel it as much. In contrast, her Eastern European patients were constantly complaining about how unbearable the pain was and how they needed more painkillers.

Pain is not merely a physiological phenomenon but also a psychological one. Thus, our attitude towards it and our mood at the time of injury may affect how painful we find it. To me, what my colleague described made sense because Eastern European cultures are, in my perception, more pessimistic and thus more attuned to negative and unpleasant emotions than the mainstream Australian culture, which tends to be cheerful. This private observation of one doctor finds its confirmation in larger research studies showing huge differences in pain perception between different ethnicities.

It is important to understand that different cultures have different health beliefs because culture can have an impact on decisions about treatment. As we live in a multicultural world, doctors may not necessarily belong to the same culture as their patients, and this can influence the advice they give. Doctors and nurses do get some training in cross-cultural issues as applied to health, but patients may never realise there may be differences in approach until there is a problem and that's why I think it is important to discuss the topic in this book.

Recently, I spent four years living in the UK and initially struggled to adjust to a different healthcare system, in particular to the way British doctors communicate – they barely speak in comparison to Australian doctors! As a person living with IBD I wanted to establish a good relationship with my GP, yet I found that GPs were not particularly interested in having a relationship with me. The expectation was that I would come to my appointment, quickly request a prescription and disappear. In my first year in the UK nobody asked how I was doing emotionally with the change of country, and nobody seemed to care at all if I was dead or alive, which was shocking to me. Luckily, I was soon referred to a friendly IBD clinic, where I established a good relationship with the IBD nurses and a specialist gastroenterologist. After trying four British GPs and finding them all uncommunicative, I decided to look for a Polish one and this person was exactly who I needed – interested in my concerns and ready to talk when I needed to discuss my worries regarding a new treatment or my wellbeing in general.

I did share my quest for a 'normal' GP with my UK colleagues at the university and they all laughed. They told me quick appointments were all they expected from their GPs. They didn't care whether it was always the same GP or a different person seeing them altogether. They wanted to spend as little time at a surgery as possible. But all these people were generally healthy and only needed to see a GP when they experienced a serious infection or had their annual check-up. When I spoke to a student of mine who had a chronic illness, she was less sanguine on the topic. She complained about too-short appointments, about doctors focusing on a single problem rather than on her overall wellbeing, about not seeing the same doctor and thus her struggle with establishing a good patient-doctor relationship. She intuitively knew she needed more from her doctor but felt powerless. There is a common perception in the UK that since healthcare is free one should not complain about it. But how else can we change it if not by discussing how to make it better (and thus noticing its faults as well as its benefits)?

So, my view is that if you don't feel you are communicating well with your GP or your specialist, find another one. While we can't immediately change the healthcare system for the better, we can look for alternatives. It is crucial to have a good relationship with your doctor, particularly if you have a long-term condition such as IBD, because if this relationship fails, and you lose confidence in your physician, you may not adhere to treatment. When we trust our doctor, we ask questions about our disease and its treatment openly and we alert the doctor to any unusual symptoms. They, on the other hand, explain what is happening, increasing our IBD knowledge and preventing any serious problems.

IBD itself varies in how it presents in different ethnicities. For example, research shows a different disease pattern in Asians with IBD from Northern Europeans – with the former having more extensive colitis but a lower risk of colectomy (a type of IBD surgery – see page 104).[3] Asian patients with Crohn's disease (CD) are also more likely to develop fistulas[4] than Hispanics and African Americans. There are many such differences and an increasing number of studies document them so that doctors know how to adjust their practice.

Culture also influences our worries in relation to IBD. For example, people in Portugal are concerned about feeling dirty or smelly due to IBD, whereas Israelis report pain and suffering as more important concerns.[5] Austrians worry about needing an ostomy bag, but not about financial implications, whereas Italians do not worry particularly about cancer due to

IBD. Caucasians fear dying from IBD complications more than African Americans, while the latter are more preoccupied with limited career choices, but also feel more stigmatised by IBD and thus talk about it less.[6]

Best practice IBD care

Long ago I promised myself that I would tell the story of my first IBD-related hospital stay if I ever got the chance, to show what healthcare should not be like, and here is my opportunity. You will know by now that I was very fortunate in getting my IBD diagnosis soon after the symptoms commenced. This was thanks to my very competent aunt, our family doctor. But my IBD diagnosis meant that I had to be transferred from my family doctor's care into the hospital system. As it was just after my seventeenth birthday, and there were no paediatric/adolescent IBD clinics in Poland at the time, I was admitted to a major adult hospital in Warsaw. To this day, the two weeks I spent there remain one of the most traumatic in my life as an IBD patient.

I shared a room with five much older ladies. One of them had suffered from CD for years and was the victim of the medical notion (popular among some doctors many years ago) that removing parts of her digestive tract one by one would cure the disease. She barely had any bowels left, and her stories of her life with IBD left me cold with dread. She had no private life, little education or work. Her whole existence centred on IBD and trying to survive. I now realise hers must have been a difficult case and with the limited treatment available then, IBD had ruined her life. I started fearing that mine might take the same turn and this made me depressed.

Opposite my bed, a lovely old lady was dying due to colorectal cancer, a complication of her long-standing IBD. She had just undergone yet another surgical procedure and was clouded by a smell of faeces. While there were other women there, these two left a vivid impression on my memory, for I imagined I would become like them, chronically disabled and eventually dying due to IBD. Initially, I slept for hours – you may remember I had an allergic reaction to sulphasalazine and was drugged with antihistamines – so I didn't have to watch IBD in its most severe form, smell it, or talk about the lives it had destroyed for a while. But then I stopped getting the anti-allergy medication and had to face the misery IBD might cause. The hospital did not offer any counselling; there was no one other than my family who would support me in dealing with the diagnosis.

The hospital where I was placed had just one bathroom for the whole ward full of women. The bathroom had two cubicles separated by a tiny wall but neither of them was fitted with a door or a curtain. Each day my mum would take up a guardian position in the door frame, her hands extended high above her head, each grabbing a corner of a large beach towel so that passers-by couldn't peek. In the cubicle next to the one I used, a generous bathtub was placed. One day when Mum and I arrived for my morning ablutions, we found a dead body there being tended by a nurse. She didn't even spare us a look. The staff were overworked, tired and indifferent to such issues as the psychological wellbeing of a patient during a hospital stay.

Interestingly, while the hospital was public, and Poland is (in theory) a non-religious country, in practice, Catholic priests had a role as second-class psychologists. This involved daily visits and aggressive persuasion to confess. *Radio Maryja* (Radio Mary), an ultra-Catholic station, played all day in the room where I stayed, and my protests against listening to *Hail, Mary* several times an hour were met with anger on the part of the overpowering priest. In his view, all Polish people were Catholic and should follow the routine he had prescribed. As I could no longer stand his visits and bathroom use was a constant stress (will there be a dead body there or not?), I begged my parents to take me home. They eventually convinced the doctor to let me go, and I visited the hospital daily for my blood tests and other examinations. I started improving as soon as I left the horrific place behind.

This story is a perfect example of a traditional approach to care, where the health practitioners are indifferent to anything beyond their individual specialist expertise. Rather than looking at a patient suffering from IBD holistically (i.e. from different angles, including physical but also psychological health), they treated the bowel, and while they did all in their power to help me battle my flare, it was in this Kafkaesque, soulless institution where I first felt truly alone.

My story also depicts a healthcare system which ignores the right of a patient to a peaceful recovery. The fact that spiritual care was enforced by priests presents another major problem. No one should be forced to follow any religious rituals, and it is even truer when one is sick and vulnerable.

The need for adolescent transition clinics

My hospital stay also demonstrates a very poor transition from paediatric to adult care. Transition means that we move from the care of our paediatric specialist to that of adult doctors. It is an important issue in IBD care. While in many cases transition is not problematic, when it goes wrong, health suffers. Flares happen during this time more often than they should, as patients may miss appointments or forget to take their medication. Hospitalisations and surgeries are more common in this period. And transition can often be stressful for patients.

Young people find it a shock as they switch from their familiar and friendly paediatric IBD clinic or their usual GP, to a more depersonalised adult service where they need to take more responsibility for their care. Not all young IBD patients are ready to move to adult clinics or be hospitalised in adult wards. Some may need time in transition care and that's why transition clinics are so important.

Quite often, the transition for an adolescent into adult IBD care occurs after a letter is sent from the paediatric gastroenterologist to the new doctor in an adult IBD service. This is a cheap method of transition, but depersonalised and capable of destroying a patient's trust in their doctor. A better model, and sufficient in 85% of patients, is a single one-hour joint clinic during which a paediatric doctor hands over care to the adult team.[7] Another, and similarly effective, option is a series of joint clinics. Permanent adolescent IBD clinics within adult hospitals can be another option, though less practical as there are very few doctors specialising in just this age group. More training for gastroenterologists may be necessary before any such initiative can become commonplace.

While my bad memories are still vivid in my head, remember this was 20 years ago, and Poland, like other countries, has greatly improved in terms of healthcare quality. IBD patients now have access to many effective treatments, such as biologics, in public hospitals. There is also good access to affordable private care as an alternative to the public system, which is famous for its long waiting times.

The role of specialist IBD clinics

Since the time of my adventures as a teenager with IBD in post-communist Poland, I have lived in two other countries and made observations on what works and what doesn't for me as a patient. The UK, for example, has specialty IBD clinics, where patients are treated by specialists rather than general practitioners. There are several clinics around the country which employ IBD nurses, who spend a much longer time with a patient than a doctor does and who provide holistic care; some clinics (though still very few) also provide access to dieticians and psychologists.

Access to IBD care nonetheless remains problematic. I hear from many UK patients that it takes a long time to be referred to a specialist, as GP care is considered cheaper than specialist care, and the focus of the National Health Service (NHS) at present is on saving money wherever possible. This was luckily not my experience, as my GP referred me to a nearby IBD clinic soon after my arrival in the UK. However, the wait to see a gastroenterologist took eight months. While waiting, I received various letters telling me that my appointment had had to be postponed (on a couple of occasions), changing dates, times and confirming all the changes (at least five letters arrived in relation to this single appointment). The most perplexing was the last letter I received shortly before my visit to the clinic. It told me to arrive on time and expect to wait several hours. It stated that while I was assigned to see a gastroenterologist it was unlikely I would see one and I would most likely see a registrar or a student. The letter ended with a caution that while I needed to allow plenty of time for my visit, there was no guarantee it would happen at all on the day I was told to report. I laughed when I read it aloud to my husband as it sounded so much like a sketch from *Little Britain*.

The care, when it eventually happened, was good, the gastroenterologist and the nurses lovely and supportive. I ended up joining a patient panel and worked with the IBD team closely. I was also offered a couple of appointments with a dietician, which helped me manage some of my symptoms, thus my long wait was worthwhile. I only worry about what would have happened to me had my IBD flared during the wait. I suspect the wait would have still been there, though possibly not as considerable as the one I endured.

The troubling aspect of care in the UK was the preoccupation with its financial side, with saving money sometimes appearing more important than providing the best care. An example of this was that sedation was not routinely offered with endoscopy. While some of us can undergo colonoscopy without sedation, many suffer during the procedure, in my opinion, unnecessarily.

For this reason, for some of the procedures I travelled to Poland where I could afford to have the procedures done in the private system without any pain or stress.

The Australian healthcare system

I am a big fan of the Australian healthcare system. To date, the care I have received in Australia for my IBD has been the best I have experienced. The system is publicly funded as in the UK, but a large proportion of the population also pay for private health insurance. There is a tax incentive to sign up for private care. What this means is that public care does not appear (to me at least) as overwhelmed as in the UK. There are waits, of course, as everywhere, but I haven't met many people with IBD (other than those based in remote areas) who could not see their gastroenterologist or their IBD nurse reasonably soon after reporting some troubling symptoms. In Australia, to shorten the waiting time, you may consider asking your GP for a permanent/ongoing referral to your gastroenterologist. That means you contact the gastroenterologist directly when you need them rather than visiting your GP first and requesting a referral each time your IBD becomes symptomatic. Scheduling check-up visits with your gastroenterologist at least once a year and ideally every six months can also help with detecting the symptoms early.

IBD nurses are becoming more and more common in IBD clinics, and while very few clinics have access to psychologists, GPs can and do refer all those who struggle psychologically for counselling, with six sessions of psychotherapy covered annually by the Australian public healthcare system (and an additional four further sessions possible in more serious cases). Isn't it the greatest place to be when one struggles with life?

Taking an integrated approach to IBD

In both Australian and UK IBD clinics, there is an increased focus on providing so-called integrated care. Integrated care is about access to a range of practitioners from different disciplines who understand IBD. Consequently, a patient receives an opinion from several specialists from disciplines such as gastroenterology, dietetics, nursing, mental health and surgery. The patient rarely sees all these people, instead meeting with the basic team (a gastroenterologist and an IBD nurse, sometimes also a psychologist) but this team communicates with other specialists on a regular basis on the patient's behalf.

Integrated care is about ongoing bio-psychosocial care (so the care is not just limited to the times of flare and encompasses not only the bowel problems but also other aspects of the illness, such as its impact on everyday life, diet, and emotional wellbeing). Good transition arrangements between paediatric and adult care are part of it as well. Crohn's & Colitis Australia's work feeds into what Australian IBD clinics do, as does that of Crohn's & Colitis UK, which feeds into the UK IBD clinics. Research is conducted on a daily basis, and the care is continuously being improved. Integrated care is recommended as current best practice by the World Health Organization. It is patient-focused, values patient views and promotes patient education. Patient panels and groups are encouraged in this model, to ensure the care is what patients need and what is best for them as per scientific evidence.

This is, of course, an ideal scenario, and not every patient experiences integrated care to the same degree. Some still complain their visits to the IBD clinic or their gastroenterologist's office are too short and leave them disappointed that their health is not being managed holistically, or that there is a lack of adequate supervision, resulting in poorer outcomes. In the past, IBD care was focused merely on addressing flares, so it was acute in nature – there was a problem prompting the doctor to act. Nowadays there is more of a focus on ongoing care – to remain healthy through prevention such as regular blood tests, a colonoscopy every few years, and ongoing medication treatment, but also addressing nutrient deficiencies and the emotional impact of IBD. The only advice I can give you if you are not satisfied with your care is to do something about it: contribute to patient surveys and patient panels, get involved in the work of patient organisations, give feedback to your IBD team and, if need be, change your doctor.

In an integrated approach to healthcare there is a role for new technologies, the internet and social media. Studies show that patients like having access to IBD-specific websites,[8] though not all existing websites would pass scrutiny by experts.[9] The websites recommended to patients are those managed by patient or doctors' organisations and are listed in the Self-help resources on page 132. New technologies are also used in some clinics to provide continuous access to care, improve patient knowledge and help self-monitor symptoms and treatment. There is increasing evidence from systematic reviews that eHealth interventions are effective and safe in managing IBD.[10]

Integrated care as a new approach to IBD is a work in progress, with very few studies evaluating its efficacy in IBD specifically (though there is plenty of research supporting it in other chronic illnesses). However, the studies that are available show that the integrated approach to care not only improves patient outcomes (e.g. reduces hospital admissions), but also results in significant savings for the healthcare system.[11] It is also appreciated by doctors.

In my own recent survey of health professionals' views on IBD care, I asked practitioners what an ideal IBD service would look like.[12] The majority would wish for easy access to integrated care, with important roles for IBD nurses, psychologists and dieticians. When I surveyed British IBD patients about their experiences with IBD care, they agreed with the doctors, that better access to dieticians and psychologists is necessary for many patients.[13] To be fair, many praised current developments in healthcare and felt their views on their IBD care were respected and valued by their IBD team, demonstrating that the move towards patient-centred care in IBD clinics has been a good one and that the care is continuously improving.

Key points

- Culture determines our beliefs and decisions in relation to health, relationships with health practitioners and attitudes towards therapy.
- If we are not aware of these differences, our communication with healthcare practitioners may suffer.
- Remember your relationship with your IBD physician is a long-term one and you should feel comfortable in it, so do not hesitate to look for a doctor whom you can trust and talk to openly.
- Some healthcare systems around the world are publicly funded, others rely on private insurance or a mixture of the two and this will mean differences in what patients experience despite best practice recommendations by the World Health Organization.
- Models of care for IBD have traditionally relied on a gastroenterologist treating a patient. Nowadays, patient-centred care is becoming the norm, where a group of knowledgeable IBD nurses, gastroenterologists, psychologists, dieticians, and surgeons share their knowledge and take a holistic approach to individual cases.
- Good transition arrangements between paediatric and adult care are important for successful long-term outcomes.
- Integrated care is appreciated by both patients and doctors and is cheaper than the traditional approach to medicine. Patients are invited to co-manage their illness, to voice their views and, as a result, care has improved.
- As a patient, knowing what best practice is currently thought to be should help you ask for what you need and work actively to improve services for yourself and others.

Chapter 8

Diagnosing IBD:
colonoscopies, endoscopies and other procedures

When I was first diagnosed with IBD I was paralysed with fear at the mere thought of undergoing a colonoscopy. I imagined it would hurt and be humiliating. This is a common anxiety. When I studied people's experiences with colonoscopy,[1] many shared my concerns. One patient summarised it beautifully by saying: 'It's a tube up your bottom; it makes people nervous.'

Many colonoscopies and gastroscopies later, I am much more sanguine on the topic. I have experienced them both under anaesthesia and without it. While I prefer to be drowsy or half asleep, the discomfort of the procedure while awake has always been manageable, at least in the case of colonoscopy. Gastroscopy (a procedure where we swallow a tube and a camera is passed down our oesophagus), while a much briefer procedure, was harder for me to tolerate awake due to my coexisting asthma. When swallowing the tube, I had a feeling I would suffocate, which I would prefer to avoid in the future. But, if you have no coexisting problems with your breathing, this procedure shouldn't bother you as much as it did me. In any case, I never found either colonoscopy or gastroscopy too painful or humiliating. They are no more so than any other medical procedures we undergo as patients with any chronic illness.

Physical examinations

However, let's start from the beginning. The most common procedure we experience during IBD treatment is physical examination. Typically, the doctor examines your abdomen by palpating it (feeling it with gentle pressure) and listening with the stethoscope. In some patients, examination of the anus and rectum is also required. This is perhaps not the pleasantest of examinations, but the doctor is usually gentle, and this examination can help in establishing if inflammation and fistulas are present.

If abscesses (swollen areas which may contain pus) are found and need to be drained, rectal examination is conducted under anaesthesia. Otherwise, physical examination is generally not painful, though it may be associated with some discomfort, and so painkillers are not offered. There is also a psychological element to it in that we are not used to showing our bare behind to strangers, so we may feel embarrassed. I can guarantee though that after a few years of living with IBD, the feeling diminishes, and we largely become indifferent. After all, we are exposing our butts in front of a medical professional and are doing so to get better. A good doctor knows you feel uncomfortable during a rectal examination and can reassure or distract you so that you are not too self-conscious.

Blood tests

After physical examination, blood tests are the second most common procedure to monitor your IBD. A needle is inserted into your vein and a small amount of blood taken. To some people, blood tests are painful. I notice that if I drink plenty of water beforehand, they don't bother me as much. If you fear the procedure, you may like to mention it to the nurse. Nurses have experience dealing with patients who are afraid of blood tests and may suggest ways to relax. Lying down and chatting to the nurse may offer enough distraction for you to forget about the pain. If the sight of the needle is what bothers you, simply look elsewhere. Some patients find it useful to bring an mp3 player and listen to music. Fortunately, blood tests don't take long and so, in the worst-case scenario, the pain lasts just seconds.

Typically, blood samples are analysed for red and white blood cell numbers and appearance, haemoglobin levels, liver function, salts and electrolytes (these can be depleted when you don't have enough fluids), vitamins such as D, folate and B12 and other parameters such as iron. Look for the ranges of these tests in the Self-help resources section on page 131. Usually, markers of inflammation such as CRP (C-reactive protein) or ESR (the erythrocyte sedimentation rate) are also examined. Blood tests are regularly repeated (sometimes every few weeks) in patients taking certain IBD medications, such as immunosuppressants. If your IBD remains in remission, you may have blood tests done annually or even less often.

Stool tests

Faecal (stool) tests are also something to be expected when you have IBD. They are commonly used to measure inflammation from stool specimens and are helpful while monitoring your disease activity. The stool tests are looking for the amounts of:

- faecal calprotectin in the stool (0–110 µg/g means the test is normal and so IBD is in remission; a value greater than 110 µg/g may indicate active IBD or other changes in the bowel such as polyps).
- lactoferrin in the stool (0–7.24 µg/ml is the normal range; 7.25 µg/ml or more indicates intestinal inflammation).

Patients are not big fans of stool tests, as nobody likes handling poo, which is smelly and disgusting. However, when you consider that faecal tests are actually the only completely pain-free procedures in IBD, they shouldn't really be dreaded. They are much less stressful than an endoscopy. If the smell is what bothers you, I find that putting a bit of Vicks VapoRub under my nose blocks it completely.

Endoscopies

An endoscopy is the general term describing different types of examinations which use a flexible tube and a camera to observe the inside of your digestive tract.

- A gastroscopy (upper endoscopy) is an examination via the mouth, reaching to your stomach and duodenum (the first part of the small intestine). It is usually a short procedure taking up to 30 minutes but typically less than that.
- A colonoscopy is an examination via the anus, up through the bowel and into the latter part of the small intestine (ileum). If the colonoscopy is focused on the lower parts of the bowel, it is called 'flexible sigmoidoscopy'. If it is focused on the rectum and anus, it is called 'proctoscopy'.

During these procedures, biopsy samples are collected. Very small pieces of the lining of your gut are gathered, and the samples obtained are then analysed. A biopsy is particularly useful in recognising if inflammation is present, establishing IBD's type and monitoring for 'dysplasia' (proliferation of abnormal cells) which is a precursor to colorectal cancer.

There is also a new type of endoscopy called 'capsule endoscopy' where, instead of the tube being inserted into your digestive tract, you swallow a small capsule containing a camera, light and recording equipment. As the capsule passes through our digestive tract, it records what it sees. This is a particularly useful tool to observe the main part of the small intestine where normal endoscopies can't reach; on the other hand, capsule endoscopies can't collect biopsies.

Quite often an endoscopy is conducted using some form of anaesthesia, as I've said, either just painkillers or also sedation which makes you drowsy. You need to fast before an endoscopy and in the case of colonoscopy, use a laxative to clear the bowel. To many patients, this is the least pleasant aspect of the procedure. Depending on the type of laxative, you may need to drink several litres of lemonade-like drink, which unfortunately is not as tasty as it sounds, and after a couple of glasses you might prefer not to drink it ever again. It makes some people nauseous, and after a few hours, urgency and bowel movements start. While sipping the laxative you should stay at home and have good access to a toilet. I usually take a day off and watch romantic comedies; I recommend similarly undemanding tasks to anyone preparing for the procedure. The colonoscopy itself takes approximately one hour, but if you have sedation you may spend several hours in hospital recovering.

Endoscopies are definitely not IBD patients' favourite procedure. We find them embarrassing and also, since our bowels are not healthy, our sensitivity to pain is heightened, particularly during flares. There is unfortunately no way to avoid an endoscopy if you have IBD, so if you are concerned, speak to your doctor or nurse to understand what happens during the procedure and request painkillers and sedation. To reassure you, studies report that the more colonoscopies we go through, the less sensitive we become to pain.[2] In addition, studies show that listening to music during colonoscopies improves patients' experience,[3] so why not bring your i-Player with you? After countless colonoscopies, the only thing I now dread is the fasting. And not because it hurts. I simply don't like being hungry!

Ultrasound, X-rays and MRI scans

Another procedure you may need to undergo is an ultrasound scan – a painless and completely harmless procedure where your insides are scanned using a sonogram (imaging based on sound waves). It is useful for uncovering changes in the abdomen, such as bowel wall thickening.

X-rays, computerised tomography (CT) and magnetic resonance imaging (MRI) are also used to establish IBD's diagnosis and monitor its extent and complications, particularly if the small intestine is involved. X-rays are usually done after swallowing a chalky liquid called a 'barium meal', which passes through the digestive tract and shows up on the resulting images. MRI and CT scans generate pictures of selected bits of the digestive tract. Of the three, only MRI does not involve radiation. Indeed, the biggest concern that patients report regarding these procedures is the long-term impact of radiation on their health. As X-rays and CT scans do slightly increase our risk of developing cancer, they are not commonly used in diagnosing IBD. Quite separately, MRI is associated with concerns about claustrophobia as you need to undergo this investigation lying in a relatively confined, enclosed tunnel. The newer machines with open sides or completely open upright ones are less problematic than the old ones, but if you are still concerned, you can always ask for sedation. The staff doing MRIs are experienced in dealing with claustrophobia. It's more common than you might think!

Key points

- The most common procedure we experience during IBD treatment is physical examination of the abdomen, anus and rectum.
- Blood tests and faecal (stool) tests are also something to be expected when you have IBD.
- Endoscopies, where a camera on a flexible tube is inserted into the gut, are of two types: a gastroscopy is an examination via the mouth that looks at the inside of the oesophagus, stomach and duodenum; a colonoscopy is an examination via the anus, that looks at the inside of the bowel and the latter part of the small intestine. They are both commonly conducted using some form of anaesthesia, either just painkillers or painkillers and sedation.
- Ultrasounds, X-rays, CT scans and MRI are other common procedures, all typically painless. As X-rays and CT scans involve radiation they are used less often but each method has particular advantages depending on what needs to be looked at.

Chapter 9

Drug treatments for IBD

Drugs are used for a number of different purposes in IBD patients:

- to suppress inflammation during a flare
- to maintain remission
- to control symptoms such as pain or diarrhoea
- to supplement nutrients.

The drugs concerned can be given as tablets, capsules, granules, injections, enemas, rectal foam or suppositories depending on the location of inflammation and the circumstances of the patient.

When you develop a bacterial infection, an antibiotic is given to kill the bacterium that is causing the infection. As we don't exactly know the cause of IBD, the available drugs cannot target this unknown factor. Instead, they target different factors which are associated with IBD. Hence, they can, for example, reduce inflammation but not its cause.

All drugs have side-effects and with every medical treatment the risks of ongoing symptoms or complications need to be weighed against the risk of possible side-effects. In this chapter I will discuss the main types of drugs used in IBD and the most common side-effects. I will not provide a full list of all side-effects as they can be easily found on the drug leaflet included in your medication box or on the internet if needed. Doctors and pharmacists can also provide you with a list of them and discuss your concerns. The overview I offer here is so you can know what to expect treatment-wise as an IBD patient.

5-aminosalicylic acid (5ASA) drugs

The 5ASAs are the most commonly used drugs in IBD. They have anti-inflammatory properties and chemically resemble aspirin. They are mostly used to maintain remission of ulcerative colitis (UC) and to lessen mild attacks of both UC and Crohn's disease (CD). Their main purpose is to lower the risk of a flare-up. They can be taken in the long term and are not considered harmful even with lifetime use.

The three commonly prescribed 5ASA drugs are sulphasalazine, olsalazine and mesalazine.

Sulphasalazine

You will recall the earlier story of my allergic reaction to sulphasalazine. While it is an effective medication, it is associated with more side-effects than the other two 5ASA drugs. If you are allergic to aspirin or sulphur antibiotics, sulphasalazin is probably not for you. If you don't know of any relevant allergy, the doctor will most likely recommend starting with a small dose just in case you are one of 10% of patients who can't tolerate it.

The most common side-effects of sulphasalazine are abdominal pain, nausea, vomiting and reduced appetite, so the doctor may recommend taking it with food. Rashes, like the one I developed when I was first diagnosed with CD, are also common, as are headaches.

Sulphasalazine can sometimes lead to male infertility, but this is reversible. However, if you are trying for a child, sulphasalazine may not be the best drug for male IBD patients. If a woman is already pregnant, sulphasalazine occasionally reduces the body's ability to absorb folic acid and she may need to supplement it. If you take sulphasalazine and notice your urine turning orange, be reassured that that's normal and not a sign of harm.

Olsalazine

Olsalazine does not have a sulphur component and that makes it suitable for people who can't tolerate sulphasalazine. It works best when the disease is located in the large intestine. Its most troubling side-effect is watery diarrhoea, and patients who experience this usually need to discontinue the drug. Olsalazine is also associated with other side-effects such as nausea, headache, abdominal pain and rashes, but luckily these are not very common (fewer than 1% of patients).

Mesalazine

Mesalazine is another alternative to sulphasalazine. This type of 5ASA is increasingly given to patients with CD (as well as UC) and is effective for mild flares and for maintaining remission, though it does not do so as effectively in CD as in UC. It is better tolerated than sulphasalazine and is rarely associated with any side-effects. However, nausea, abdominal pain, rashes and headaches can occasionally occur.

Mesalazine is the most universal of the 5ASA drugs as it comes in several formulations targeting different parts of the digestive tract; some work best for the last part of the small intestine (ileum) and the beginning of the colon; others are focused on the large intestine, but there are also some which work throughout the gut.

Mesalazine is available as tablets, granules, enemas (a liquid injection into the rectum), foams (similar to enemas but in the form of foams rather than liquids) and suppositories (solid, often bullet-shaped, preparations to be inserted via the rectum). The three latter are used if IBD is limited to the lower part of the bowel, while the tablets and granules are given if IBD is located in the upper parts of the bowel. These delivery methods have the advantage that the drug can be delivered directly to the affected part of the bowel. The drug is not absorbed into the blood and as a result presents with practically no side-effects. Suppositories are only helpful if your IBD is confined to the rectum.

Corticosteroids (steroids)

Steroids are used to treat acute attacks of IBD. They are like cortisol, which is a hormone naturally produced by the human body. They work on the immune system and block inflammatory responses, thus reducing swelling and pain. Steroids work fast, and you will notice an improvement within days of starting the therapy.

They can be given as tablets, enemas, foams, suppositories or intravenous injections. Tablets and injections reduce inflammation throughout the body and so, if you have 'extra-intestinal' symptoms of IBD, such as inflammation in the eyes or joints, steroids will take care of them too. Rectal steroids given as enemas are effective when disease is limited to the large bowel and they then produce fewer side-effects than when given orally or intravenously (into a vein). Most commonly, however, steroids are given orally, and they are famous for their side-effects; consequently they are not prescribed for long periods of time. Typically, the doctor will recommend a high dose for a short time and then a slow withdrawal over several weeks. Steroids cannot be stopped suddenly because, when we take high doses, our body stops producing its own and it needs to be given the time to take this function over again, otherwise patients are likely to experience some unpleasant symptoms, such as agitation, nausea, fatigue and light-headedness. In some people, even sudden drops in dose may result in these effects; thus you should really be weaned off them slowly.

The most common side-effect of steroids is increased appetite and weight gain, with common features being a 'moon face' and 'buffalo hump' (when fat develops in the middle of the upper back). Other possible effects include acne, facial hair, easy bruising and swollen ankles. Mood changes also often occur, and these can include agitation, irritability or depression. Importantly, steroids remove the body's natural protection against infections, with healing becoming impaired. They raise blood sugar levels and, taken in the long term, may lead to diabetes. They can also raise blood pressure.

In children, as mentioned in Chapter 4, they halt growth. However, children with active IBD do not grow or develop normally anyway, so it is better to focus on healing inflammation as the priority. After a child's IBD has improved, their development usually gets back to normal.

There are also side-effects which, unlike those mentioned so far, are irreversible. Cataracts and bone damage are the most significant, with the latter leading to osteoporosis. They tend to occur with long-term steroid treatment in people with other risk factors, such as in post-menopausal women.

As you can see, steroids are not 'a piece of cake', but to balance all this negativity, after weeks or months of horrible symptoms, many IBD patients who start taking steroids finally feel normal again. Steroids give you energy and the day when you go to the loo just once (as opposed to 15 or 20 times during your flare), and your bowel movement is back to normal, feels like the best day of your life. For most patients I know, steroids are worth the downside as they may mean weeks, months or even years of being healthy.

Common types of steroids are prednisolone, prednisone and hydrocortisone. Most recently, budesonide has been used in IBD. It is a newer kind of steroid which is not associated with as many side-effects as the old types. It is mostly used in CD when the end of the small intestine and the beginning of the bowel are affected. Beclometasone dipropionate (also known as BDP or Clipper) is an alternative to older steroids for UC patients. If you are concerned about being given one of the older steroids, ask your doctor whether any of these two newer ones are an option for you.

Immunosuppressants

Immunosuppressants (they suppress your immune system, meaning that they weaken its response) are used when 5ASA and steroids have failed or when a patient becomes dependent on steroids and withdrawal from them causes a flare. They are thus given in cases of IBD which are hard to control. They are similar to steroids in that they act on the immune system, suppressing its activity and thus reducing inflammation. They were originally developed to help people after transplants and in cancer treatment. The most commonly used in IBD are the thiopurines.

Thiopurines: azathioprine and mercaptopurine (or 6-MP)

The thiopurines azathioprine and mercaptopurine (otherwise known as 6-MP) are the most commonly used immunosuppressants in IBD. They are both available as tablets. They control both CD and UC and prevent flares in both diseases but are less commonly used to treat UC as UC can be better managed through surgery. It takes quite a long time, often up to six months, for the drug to start working. The most significant side-effect is the increase in chance of infection with 'flu or a cold, for example, as azathioprine reduces white cell production. If you are prescribed this drug, you will have regular blood tests and will be monitored for any signs of infection. Other side-effects include nausea, loss of appetite, fever, rashes and inflammation of the liver or pancreas. While taking these drugs, one's skin becomes sensitive to sunlight and thus direct exposure needs to be avoided and sunblock applied as there is an increased risk of skin cancer. Unlike steroids, azathioprine and 6-MP can be stopped immediately.

Methotrexate

Methotrexate was developed as a treatment for cancer and, in the IBD context, is mostly used in CD during flares, to induce remission, and then to maintain it. Like azathioprine and 6-MP, it is given to people who are steroid-dependent, but it can be an alternative for those who cannot tolerate either of those drugs. It is taken once a week and can be given as a tablet or injection. It takes up to three months to start working. Like the other immunosuppressants, it makes one more prone to infections and more sensitive to sunlight. Nausea and diarrhoea at the beginning of treatment are also relatively common. Liver and kidney problems may occur, and thus regular blood tests are a must.

If you are a woman, you shouldn't become pregnant while you or your partner are taking methotrexate. It can have serious effects on the unborn baby. It is recommended to stop taking methotrexate three to six months before trying to conceive.

Cyclosporine

Cyclosporine is often used in people after they have received an organ transplant. In UC, it may help you avoid surgery. It can be a useful addition to azathioprine as it starts working faster while azathioprine needs several months to take effect. Cyclosporine is usually given by injection at a hospital, but may also be given orally and is typically recommended for three to six months.

It is associated with many side-effects, including susceptibility to infection, nausea, high blood pressure, impaired kidney function, facial hair growth, gum swelling and pins and needles in the fingers and toes. Regular blood tests are needed, particularly to monitor kidney function.

Tacrolimus and mycophenolate mofetil

These two drugs are used less commonly than the other immunosuppressants described above. Tacrolimus resembles cyclosporine but may be used for severe CD as well as for UC. Like cyclosporine, it is often given with azathioprine whilst waiting for the latter drug to become effective. It can be taken orally and as an ointment when IBD is located in the anal area and rectum. Side-effects are similar to cyclosporine.

Mycophenolate mofetil has been used to treat cancer and to support organ transplants. In IBD, it is used in patients who do not respond well to other immunosuppressants or biologics.

Biologics

Biologics are the newest IBD treatment. They work by reducing the amount of an immune mediator of IBD, a protein called TNF-alpha which is overproduced when IBD inflammation occurs. They are made from substances which occur in nature and are produced using a biological rather than chemical process. They can come from a living cell – for example, from mouse tissue. Biologics are prescribed for severe IBD when other treatments have not worked. Blood tests to monitor your health are used similarly to immunosuppressants. The most commonly prescribed is infliximab.

Infliximab

If you have severe CD or UC and haven't responded to steroids or immunosuppressants, you are likely to be prescribed infliximab. For some patients, it can be very effective in bringing about remission and reducing the need for surgery. It is given in hospital intravenously (into a vein – a drip lasting two hours). After the first dose, another is given two weeks later and then another after six to eight weeks.

Before you start taking infliximab it's important to undergo a test for tuberculosis as infliximab can reactivate it; it is also important to tell your doctor about all other infections (fungal, bacterial, etc) you have had recently. Side-effects include susceptibility to infections, nausea, headache, stomach pain, rashes, and possibly a worsening of a pre-existing heart condition. More rarely, liver or nervous system problems occur.

Adalimumab

Adalimumab is typically used for controlling flares and fistulas in severe CD or when a patient has not responded to infliximab. It's injected under the skin (so not into a vein). Side-effects are similar to those for infliximab but another adalimumab-specific common side-effect is pain at the injection site.

Importantly, while side-effects can occur with anti-TNF alpha treatment, many patients do not report them or report only minor and temporary ones so we can assume it is largely side-effect-free. At the same time, there is good evidence that these drugs significantly improve quality of life.

Other biologics

There are two other biologics which you may encounter during your treatment for IBD. They are newer than the previously discussed treatments, hence you may only hear about them in the future. Golimumab is used in adults with UC who have not responded to, or been able to tolerate, other treatments.

Vedolizumab is used in both UC and CD and, similarly to golimumab, is used if a patient has had problems with other treatments.

Other drugs

Anti-diarrhoaeals

Anti-diarrhoaeals slow down muscle activity in the gut, which allows the water produced during digestion to be reabsorbed by the colon, resulting in firmer stools and less urgency to defaecate. For IBD patients, the safest anti-diarrhoeal is loperamide; however, it does produce some side-effects. It may result in constipation and hard stools which are difficult to pass.

Anti-diarrhoeals are not recommended during UC flares as they may result in a blockage.

Laxatives

In some instances, for example when IBD is located in the rectum, constipation may be a symptom. In such cases, laxatives can be used. Laxatives make the stools softer by increasing the amount of water in the bowel. It is important that the laxatives you take contain a compound called macrogol which is suitable for IBD. Their side-effects include wind and cramps.

Anti-spasmodics

Anti-spasmodics reduce painful gut cramps or spasms by relaxing the intestinal muscles. They may be useful if you have so-called 'IBS in IBD' (see Chapter 1, page 11). Examples include mebeverine, hyoscine butylbromide and alverine citrate. They are generally safe, and don't produce many side-effects, although in some people temporary blurred vision may occasionally occur which affects the ability to drive.

Bile-salt binders

If you suffer from CD and have had your ileum (the latter part of your small intestine) removed, higher levels of bile salts (naturally produced by the liver) as a consequence of the surgery, can lead to diarrhoea. Bile-salt binders include cholestyramine, colestipol and colesevalam. They prevent the bile salts from reaching the colon, thus stopping the diarrhoea from developing. They are available as a powder (cholestryramine and colestipol) which can be mixed with drinks or food, or as tablets (colesevalam).

Side-effects include indigestion, bloating and abdominal discomfort, nausea and constipation. You need to make sure that you don't take them at the same time of day as other drugs as they affect how other drugs are absorbed. It's best to wait four hours after having bile-salt binders before taking other medication.

Bulking agents

If you've undergone surgery to remove your colon (colectomy), diarrhoea may be a consequence and bulking agents have been found useful in controlling it in these circumstances. They can also help with constipation resulting from IBD located in the rectum. These medications contain a water-absorbent plant fibre and are available as granules which need to be taken with water. They swell up inside your bowel, thickening liquid or softening hard stools. They are generally safe but shouldn't be taken if you have CD with a narrowing of the bowel (stricture).

Antibiotics

Metronidazole and ciprofloxacin may be helpful for treating active CD and may help after surgery.

Metronidazole is used in CD when abscesses or fistulas are present and has a beneficial effect on the large bowel. The most common side-effects are nausea and loss of appetite. Other side-effects include indigestion, diarrhoea and headaches. Importantly, you should not drink alcohol when taking metronidazole as the two may interact producing unpleasant symptoms such as palpitations, nausea, shortness of breath and drowsiness.

Ciprofloxacin has fewer side-effects than metronidazole. It is normally taken as a tablet but can be given by injection as well. Common side-effects include nausea and diarrhoea. However, ciprofloxacin may interact with some of the other IBD medications and thus you may be prescribed metronidazole.

Painkillers

Pain is a common symptom in IBD. The best treatment for IBD-related pain is to get rid of inflammation, but as that may take some time to achieve, some patients take painkillers. Paracetamol or paracetamol-with-codeine are the safest options in IBD. They should not be taken for a long period, though.

Aspirin, ibuprofen and diclofenac should be avoided as they are known to aggravate the symptoms of IBD and may even trigger an IBD flare. Be mindful of which painkillers you reach for!

Vitamins and minerals

Some patients with CD require regular injections of vitamin B12, which is essential for nerve and brain functions. It is absorbed from the lower part of the small bowel – the ileum – and, if this is affected by IBD or has been removed surgically, B12 absorption can be impaired. B12 is typically given by injection every three months. If the ileum has been removed these injections will be needed for life.

In some patients, particularly those losing a lot of blood during bowel movements, iron and folic acid deficiencies occur and these then need to be supplemented. Iron changes the colour of your stool to black, so don't freak out if you spot dark wastes in your toilet bowl after taking it. Indigestion and nausea are common side-effects. Be aware that taking folic acid (vitamin B9) as a supplement will disguise the effects of vitamin B12 deficiency on a blood sample – make sure any health professional testing for B12 deficiency is aware of this.

For those CD patients who have problems absorbing fat, supplementation with fat-soluble vitamins (i.e. A, D, E and K) may also be necessary.

Medication compliance

IBD is a chronic condition, so it is unlikely suddenly to disappear from your life. We know that some medications can prolong the periods of remission, but for the medication to have this effect it needs to be taken regularly and even if symptoms are not problematic or have disappeared completely. Quite often, patients who have just been diagnosed with IBD and have debilitating symptoms take their medication religiously. But as soon as the symptoms settle down, we all feel tempted to reduce the dose or forget about it altogether. Unfortunately, as we have been 'blessed' with a chronic illness, we need to take the medication continuously to reduce the chance of a flare. If we stick to this routine, it is likely that when the next flare comes it will be easier to manage. Continuous treatment also protects us from other conditions – for example, 5ASAs have a protective effect against bowel cancer in people with IBD, so it's worth persevering with the treatment.

There is no need to panic if you forget to take a dose occasionally, but if you stop taking the medication completely or remember about it only once a week, you will lose the protection. It's worth speaking to your IBD nurse or doctor if you struggle with maintaining the routine. They will give you advice on how not to forget. This may include taking medication at the time when you brush your teeth or with a meal, for example.

Studies show that mental state, and depression in particular, affect compliance with treatment[1] and that's yet another reason to seek help if we feel overwhelmed by IBD or life in general. Another important issue influencing compliance with treatment is the relationship with your doctor. When this relationship is not transparent, supportive, respectful and based on empathy, IBD patients are more likely to stop being compliant with treatment.[2] As I have said in Chapter 7, and elsewhere in this book, if you don't trust your IBD doctor, it may be the time to look for another. After all, you wouldn't accept a friend or a spouse who you don't trust, so why have such a doctor? Your health is at stake here!

Antidepressants

This is a good point at which to discuss the use of antidepressants. My interest in antidepressants started in 2004. Despite having graduated from two prestigious Polish universities, I struggled with securing a job in Poland, so I decided I would pursue a doctorate. I wasn't certain in what area, as I had many research interests, from cognitive psychology to international politics, and thus I explored different options. At around this time, my then boyfriend, who has since become my husband, had the brilliant idea of moving to the Antipodes to see what life tasted like Down Under. I only needed to come up with a research idea to secure a PhD scholarship which would grant us both a visa and we could then sample what Australia had to offer.

My PhD topic came to me in a dream, or perhaps it was a daydream? I can't remember exactly, but I know that my subconscious played a part. At that time, I had never considered IBD as a strong research interest. It was a disease I had, and something I tried not to think too much about for, as it was, it took plenty of my life and willpower in frequent visits to doctors, treatment side-effects and toilet dependence. Therefore, IBD wasn't among the topics I was reading up on when searching for a good PhD idea. But it did make sense. The dream wasn't an elaborate one. It simply showed myself sitting in bed and daydreaming – so a dream within a dream. My day-dreaming self wondered: since people with IBD often get diarrhoea when stressed, would giving them antidepressants stop it? It was that simple. I then started looking for the answer to my question and found that nobody had studied the role of antidepressants in IBD. I thought I would, as this was a question to which I wanted to know the answer for myself. Here my adventure as an IBD scientist started, coincidentally, in the continent in which antidepressants were first trialled in psychiatric practice.

Antidepressants are a twentieth-century phenomenon. While lithium, one of the first antidepressants, was known in the nineteenth century, it was introduced to psychiatry practice around the 1950s. Its contemporary history starts in Melbourne, Australia, when John Cade used it to treat mania. His experiment was later repeated by C.H. Noack and E.M. Trautner, also from Melbourne, who examined the use of lithium in 100 patients and concluded that its benefits much outweighed the risks. It has since been used for many different psychiatric conditions, including depression and bipolar disorder; however, it has been systematically replaced by newer and safer drugs.

Tricyclic antidepressants also entered the market in the 1950s and quickly became the first choice for treating depression. Interestingly, they have been widely used in gastroenterology, mainly to manage IBS (see Chapter 1). IBS can be hard to treat and involves a significant psychological component. Because the psychology of the patient has long been considered important in IBS, antidepressants have been proposed as one of the treatments. There is good evidence from systematic reviews that tricyclic antidepressants can improve bowel functions (i.e. can reduce diarrhoea) and help with bowel pain.[3, 4]

The most commonly used antidepressants nowadays are SSRIs (selective serotonin reuptake inhibitors) which were introduced in the 1980s. The best known of them is fluoxetine. They are considered safer than tricyclic antidepressants, yet still can cause side-effects, such as drowsiness, dry mouth, insomnia, dizziness, nervousness and sexual problems. From the point of view of the digestive system, they may cause gastrointestinal dysfunction (nausea, diarrhoea, stomach pain) in the first weeks of taking them, but high quality systematic reviews (the gold standard for drug research) consider them equally effective in patients with IBS as the tricyclics.[3, 4]

There are also other types of antidepressant that don't fit within the above-mentioned groups and which are used in patients with bowel problems, but there is less evidence regarding their efficacy. For example, there are some early encouraging data on the usefulness of mirtazapine, which is a tetracyclic antidepressant particularly useful in patients who suffer from nausea and poor appetite, and on duloxetine which is an SNRI (serotonin norepinephrine reuptake inhibitor) antidepressant particularly effective for pain.[5]

You may have noticed that while these drugs have been designed as treatment for mental disorders, they have many other uses. For depression, there has long been a controversy regarding their efficacy. While they help for severe mental illness, their effect in mild depression is questionable.[6]

What interested me, however, was whether they can help IBD by reducing either diarrhoea, pain or inflammation. From a systematic review of the role of antidepressants in depression associated with chronic illness,[7] I learnt that they are effective in treating depression in people who are physically ill. Some studies have shown that antidepressants have anti-inflammatory properties, and thus, for example, people suffering from asthma who take antidepressants don't need as much of their steroid medication. But how does it look in IBD? Is there any benefit in taking antidepressants?

The answer is not simple as there have been very few good

quality studies. We know that a significant proportion of IBD patients take antidepressants (up to 30%), with those patients with more severe IBD taking them more commonly.[8, 9] We know that many of these patients don't have depression, anxiety or high levels of stress, and thus they seem to be being prescribed antidepressants specifically for the symptoms of IBD.

What would happen if an IBD patient without depression took antidepressants? Most likely their IBD symptoms would slightly improve.

I conducted three systematic reviews in the area. (I have explained what these are in the Preface (page xvi).) The first one, now 10 years old, identified 12 studies, all of them in humans, relatively small-scale and none of them experimental. (Only 'experimental studies' can tell us if a particular treatment is effective for IBD; 'observational studies' merely observe people taking antidepressants but can't tell us if the effect is due to antidepressants or other factors.) These studies suggested some benefit from antidepressants for both mental and physical health in IBD.[10]

The second review was focused on animal research.[11] There have been quite a number of animal studies in which mice or rats with colitis were given antidepressants and their colitis healed. These findings were encouraging but, as scientists well know, the fact that something works in animals doesn't mean the same will be true in humans.

Most recently, together with a group of colleagues, I conducted a third systematic review.[12] There have been a few new studies, but still not many, with 15 in total included in the review. Most concluded that antidepressants had a beneficial effect on the course of IBD and improved anxiety and depression, which was encouraging. However, since we are talking here about a small number of studies of moderate quality, I think we need to wait a few years before we can recommend antidepressants as an adjuvant treatment for IBD to be prescribed together with 5ASA drugs and biologics. It is also uncertain which antidepressants should be recommended, as the studies varied in their findings. Watch this space.

Key points

- Medication in IBD is used to suppress inflammation during a flare; to maintain remission; to control symptoms such as pain or diarrhoea; and to provide nutrients.
- The 5ASAs are the most commonly used drugs in IBD. They maintain remission of UC and are prescribed in mild attacks of both UC and CD.
- Corticosteroids are used to treat acute attacks of IBD. Steroids work fast, and you will notice improvement within days of starting the therapy. They are known for their side-effects and generally are prescribed for short periods of time.
- Immunosuppressants are used when 5ASA and steroids have failed, or when the person with IBD becomes dependent on steroids and withdrawal from them causes a flare. They take several months to work, and their main side-effect is increasing the likelihood of infections.
- Biologics are the newest type of treatment for IBD. Biologics are prescribed for severe IBD when other treatments have not worked.
- Anti-diarrhoeals are commonly used in IBD to control urgency and dehydration but are not recommended during UC flares as they may result in blockages.
- Laxatives are used to help with constipation and make the stools softer by increasing the amount of water in the bowel.
- Anti-spasmodics reduce painful gut cramps or spasms.
- Bile-salt binders are used in CD when the ileum has been removed in part or in full; they help manage the diarrhoea that arises from that.
- Bulking agents are another type of treatment, used after colectomy (removal of part of the colon); they help with both diarrhoea and constipation.
- Certain antibiotics may be helpful in treating active CD and also help after surgery.
- Vitamin and mineral supplementation, such as with B12 or iron, is often needed in IBD.

- Compliance with IBD treatment is essential to manage the disease and improve quality of life, but also to prevent colorectal cancer. Mental illness and poor patient-doctor relationships are common reasons for medication non-adherence.
- Antidepressants are nowadays used not only to treat depression but also to help with physical symptoms, such as pain and insomnia.
- A group of antidepressants called tricyclics have been used for quite a while to help with bowel symptoms in functional gut disorders, such as IBS and dyspepsia (chronic 'indigestion').
- Newer groups of antidepressants – SSRIs and SNRIs – have also been found helpful for bowel symptoms.
- Some antidepressants have been found to have anti-inflammatory properties.
- Studies in people with IBD taking antidepressants are limited, but the current evidence is encouraging, showing improvements in bowel symptoms.

Chapter 10

Surgery and IBD

Many IBD patients fear surgery. The picture that springs to mind as soon as the doctor mentions an operation for IBD is an ostomy bag (i.e. a small plastic pouch worn over a stoma to collect stool). Studies show this to be one of the top fears of IBD patients. The prospect of carrying your poo in a bag with you wherever you go is not a particularly attractive one. What if the bag breaks while you are in company, spilling its smelly contents? And, to dig deeper, what does the need for surgery mean about me as a patient? Am I so sick that I require an invasive procedure? What about post-operative pain and recovery? And what's the likelihood that it won't help? Because of these fears, surgery is often considered by people living with IBD to be the last resort, to be avoided at all cost.

Surgery, in general, is not something one looks forward to, whether you suffer from IBD or not. It is by no means pleasant. Lying in a hospital bed, attached to various pieces of medical equipment, inhaling the bleachy scent of hospital disinfectants, we are at our most vulnerable. We feel out of control and completely reliant on doctors, nurses and our loved ones. If we have no previous experience, surgery is an unknown and as any unknown it creates uncertainty. If we've had a surgery before and it didn't go well, we expect the next one will be as horrible as the last one. But even being hospitalised for IBD (without surgery) is associated with significant anxiety and can have lasting impact on mental health.[1] Hence, part of the fear of having a surgery is a fear of being hospitalised.

As a person who has experienced two keyhole (i.e. laparoscopic) procedures to my abdomen, I can attest to all such fears being, to some degree, justified. However, before the surgery, when we worry and anticipate all possible perils, we generally overestimate its unpleasant aspects. Recovery is rarely as slow and as painful as we first imagine. In modern surgical practice, doctors encourage patients to return to normal life as soon as possible, and there are effective medications to support one's recovery.

After my first surgery, I was shocked that the nurse asked me to stand up from my bed and walk as soon as the very next morning. My tummy was swollen, the wound still fresh and I felt lightheaded. At least the pain wasn't there, as I was heavily drugged. I don't have fond memories of the first night after that operation – I was nauseous and vomited after the anaesthetics, and I was asked to lie down without being allowed to move much. But you will laugh when I tell you that my greatest fear was not about whether the surgery would be successful, or even whether I would be in pain. It was about having to have the catheter attached to my urethra. For some reason, the thought of that terrified me most. Quite unnecessarily, as the little tube was put in after I fell asleep and its removal didn't hurt a bit.

Beyond that first night, I don't have any difficult memories. I'm sure there were times when my tummy felt uncomfortable, when my stitches turned itchy, or I was exhausted, but all these feelings were manageable and have dimmed in my memory over time. Both my operations were minimally invasive and successful and that may, of course, influence my positive recollection of them, but I think what also helped was that I spent some time speaking to my doctor – a person I trust – about the pros and cons of the surgery, and that I discussed the sedation (this involved a general anaesthetic with intubation, which I was concerned about) with an anaesthetist (a doctor who manages your pain during a surgery). The support of my family and friends meant that I could also focus on recovering rather than worrying about other things, such as cooking or cleaning the house. So, if I was to give advice based on my experience, I would recommend improving your knowledge of the surgery – what it involves, its risks but also its benefits for your quality of life – and giving yourself the time to consider this as compared with other options, and seeking support from your nearest and dearest.

How common is it to need surgery in IBD?

The numbers of people requiring surgery in both UC and CD have decreased quite substantially over the last decades.[2] While in the past it could be as high as 70–90% in CD, at present, in CD, one year post-diagnosis it is 16%, five years post-diagnosis it is 33%, and 10 years post-diagnosis it is 46%. In UC it is 5%, 12% and 16%, respectively.[2]

While in CD the most common type of surgery is resection (i.e. cutting out part of the intestines), a colectomy (a removal of the colon/large bowel) of some type is usually conducted in UC. Studies have shown that total abdominal colectomy with end ileostomy (so, removal of the colon and creation of a stoma) is a safe procedure. This doesn't mean there are no complications. In fact, up to 30% of patients experience some complications (e.g. infections), but mortality in patients whose bowel was not perforated (bowel perforation is very dangerous and increases the risk of mortality) is very low (0%–4%).

Does surgery work?

The statistics are indeed reassuring, showing that IBD surgery is largely successful.[3, 4] What is more, surgery can be a permanent cure for UC and can induce remission in CD. So, while weighing our options, we need to remember there is potentially a lot to gain from surgery. Patients often mention complications and adverse events associated with surgical procedures, forgetting that their usual IBD treatments have side-effects as well (see Chapter 9). With all IBD treatment, it is always about considering pros and cons, and coming up with what is more acceptable to us than the alternative.

In my clinical and research work, I have met quite a few patients with UC who couldn't praise surgery enough and only regretted they had suffered the symptoms so long instead of agreeing to have it done when this option had been first offered to them. Research confirms that quality of life improves after surgery,[5] sometimes not straight away (we need to recover first), but long-term quality of life after surgery is better than before the operation and comparable to that in the general population (i.e. healthy people).[6] On the other hand, surgery is also linked in some studies to the risk of anxiety and depression, with up to 15% of patients being diagnosed with anxiety and/or depression within five years post-surgery; this is particularly the case in those who have surgery early on in life. Thus, while surgery can be a life changer in some (particularly UC) patients, it does affect others (though very few) less positively.

Do you always have to have an ostomy bag?

And what about the feared ostomy bag? First, not all surgical procedures done in IBD involve creating a stoma (i.e. a hole in the abdomen where a bag can be attached to collect faecal matter). In fact, only a small percentage of patients need a stoma, and in an even smaller number of people a stoma is a permanent fixture. But, of course, when a stoma needs to be created we know that in the short term it can affect your quality of life, and not for the better. The potential leakage and ballooning of bags does affect one's self-confidence and can lead to social isolation.[7] The surgery also has an impact on our sexual lives, partly due to our self-image being negatively affected and partly for practical reasons – it takes a while to figure out what to do with an ostomy bag during intercourse. While not many studies have been conducted in this area, it appears that in the long term, people adapt to living with a stoma and their quality of life improves.[8, 9] A good relationship with your doctor and a stoma nurse in whom you can confide your problems and discuss issues such as lower libido post-surgery, can help speed up the adjustment to having a stoma.[9] As always, open communication with your partner is essential. Inviting them to your doctor's or nurse's appointment to discuss adjustments to your life may help both you and them in coping with this change.

Of interest to those who fear the ostomy bag, there is an alternative. Proctocolectomy with ileal pouch-anal anastomosis (IPAA) is the most commonly performed procedure in UC nowadays, and it does not require wearing an ostomy bag permanently. During this surgery, the colon and the rectum are removed, but the anus and some muscles are preserved. The ileum (the lower portion of the small intestine) is then shaped into a pouch (sometimes called the 'J pouch') and connected to the anus. The pouch stores the waste material until you defaecate. Because the pouch needs to heal, a temporary ileostomy (i.e. a hole in the abdomen for the elimination of waste) is created and the bag temporarily attached to it. After approximately 12 weeks, another smaller operation is performed, and the temporary ileostomy closed, and thus an ostomy bag is no longer required. Unfortunately, this type of surgery has a slightly higher complications rate than total colectomy.[10]

Your colorectal surgeon or gastroenterologist will be able to tell you whether your disease type and your other characteristics predispose you to respond well to surgery and which procedure might be appropriate. While I hope you will not need it, remember that when you do, surgeries of the bowel are common and safe procedures which can potentially improve your life. Their risks and benefits need to be weighed up, but that's true for any treatment, and your doctor should be able to help you make an informed decision.

Key points

- Surgery for IBD is one of the greatest fears of people living with IBD, yet studies show that IBD surgery is usually safe and largely successful, and that quality of life improves in the long term post-surgery.
- Short-term problems with stomas, such as leakage and ballooning of bags, may lead to social isolation. In addition, anxiety and depression may develop after surgery, particularly in young patients. Therefore, if you notice that your mood deteriorates post-surgery, speak to your doctor and seek a referral to a mental health specialist.
- As for any treatment, risks and benefits need to be weighed up. A good relationship with your doctor and stoma nurse is crucial for your recovery and addressing any concerns.

Chapter 11

The role of diet and exercise

Diet

They say you are what you eat. The most obvious solution that comes to mind when one is diagnosed with a gastrointestinal condition is therefore to change your diet. But will any specific diet cure IBD? The answer is a straight no. There is no scientific evidence for it. We cannot cure IBD by switching to organic food, avoiding food colourants or preservatives or adopting any special diet. But, and it's an important but, we can reduce some of the symptoms of IBD, address nutritional deficits (lack of certain vitamins, for example), maintain healthy body weight and, as a result, feel better by adjusting what we eat.

IBD patients often observe that some foods make their IBD worse. Lactose sensitivity (being able to tolerate only small quantities of products that include lactose, such as cow's milk) or intolerance (can't tolerate lactose at all) is often reported by IBD patients. Saturated fat and fatty dishes (e.g. those including butter, mayonnaise or fried food) can cause problems. Sweeteners are often another no-no food (e.g. aspartame, included in soft drinks and some chewing gums). Chocolate, coffee and nuts are often avoided. Some vegetables, such as beans, cabbage and broccoli, but also onion, may cause problems. Spicy food (e.g. dishes including chilli) can also make the symptoms worse, as may apparently healthy choices, such as whole grains.

What is there left that you can eat, you may well ask? The good news is that all these foods are rarely bad for you at the same time. Sometimes, it's just one of them. I was seeing a patient a few years ago whose symptoms improved dramatically when he removed onion from his diet. Just onion, though it took him a while to discover that many ready-made sauces he used included it, so he had to start cooking more for himself. I met another patient who, while in remission, suffered diarrhoea 10 times a day but whose bowel symptoms ceased to bother him the moment he stopped drinking diet coke (which included a sweetener). He drank two litres of it a day believing it was better for him than regular coke. Whether two litres of coke (of any type) can be good for anyone is questionable, but the choice this person had made was devastating to his bowel as sweeteners, particularly in large quantities, lead to diarrhoea.

Talking to many patients who participated in my own research studies and those who I have met through my psychological work, there is no universal intolerance to one type of food. Some of us drink cow's milk, eat chips and chocolate and don't feel any worse. Thus, the important thing about diet in IBD is self-awareness. You need to experiment and see what works and what doesn't for you. There is no way of avoiding it. Usually, soon after the diagnosis is made or even before, you will notice you suffer diarrhoea or bloating after some products and can adjust your diet accordingly through trial and error. If you are only now learning you have IBD and feel exasperated about your diet, be assured it gets easier. After some time, you will know what you can eat and what you need to avoid.

When my IBD started I suddenly became allergic to mushrooms, which I had eaten without any problems till then. I am talking about allergy rather than intolerance as the symptoms are not merely unpleasant but also potentially life-threatening – a high fever, vomiting, difficulty breathing and a rash. I have since avoided mushrooms. In Poland, where many types of mushroom are eaten all year round but particularly at Christmas, I had to leave home when they were being prepared as even the smell of mushrooms being baked in the oven triggered a reaction.

Interestingly, our tolerance of some foods may change over time, and some products may only affect you during flares while others will be on a ban list permanently. In my case, what changed was my tolerance of meat, which has diminished quite significantly since my diagnosis. At present I can only tolerate poultry, some seafood and occasionally beef. I can't eat pork – even a tiny bite of it causes problems. The last time I ate a bit of a sausage, several years ago, I was sick for three days. Other red meats are also not good for me and even the lean beef I occasionally have I can tolerate only in very small quantities. Yet, a fully vegetarian diet did not serve me either. Despite my attempts to keep up my iron and B12, a vegetarian diet left me anaemic. As I can't tolerate many of the healthy sources of these nutrients, I take regular supplementation and make myself eat beef occasionally.

It is important to see a dietician at least once about your diet and IBD. Only a few IBD clinics worldwide offer this service and, if your clinic does, I cannot recommend it highly enough. The dietician should ideally know about current practice in IBD and most importantly understand that the normal healthy diet principles (i.e. eat a lot of fibre and wholegrains) may not apply in IBD. The first time I spoke to a dietician about my diet and IBD, I was told my diet was too healthy! My multigrain dark bread was replaced with a white flour bun. Veggies such as lentils and broccoli, which I enjoyed daily, were to be limited, while avocado, corn and raspberries were best completely forgotten. The plus of this dietary approach was that I found that some of the foods needed to be eliminated only for a few weeks and could be reintroduced slowly.

What does science tell us about diet in IBD? A healthy IBD

diet is about ensuring healthy nutritional status. Malnutrition is common in children with IBD, and good diet is essential to support growth. Osteoporosis is a common side-effect of some of IBD treatments, and the right diet can prevent it. Many patients, particularly those suffering from Crohn's disease (CD), are underweight and malnourished. When IBD flares, we don't feel like eating and the inflammation and fever make our body burn calories faster, which contributes to weight loss. Even when weight loss is not a concern, good nutrition is paramount for keeping healthy.

Common nutritional problems in IBD include low iron, folate and B12, but also deficiencies in other vitamins (e.g. vitamin D) and minerals (e.g. calcium, selenium and zinc, which happen to be essential for maintaining good mental health). Problems with digesting fat (even healthy fats) are common, as are low levels of electrolytes (mostly due to diarrhoea and a too low fluid intake – 2 litres of fluid a day are necessary in healthy people).[1] While not all people living with IBD need vitamin and mineral supplementation, those suffering long flares, taking steroids or sulphasalazine, after resection, and those suffering excessive diarrhoea usually require some help with their nutrients.

Probiotics such as lactobacilli and bifidobacteria (see Chapter 2) may also be helpful in IBD, particularly in ulcerative colitis (UC), where products such as VSL#3 support maintenance of remission.[2] Unfortunately, there is no evidence that VSL#3 helps CD. While we know IBD is very much about an inappropriate response to gut bacteria, we cannot be sure which probiotics are best for repairing the faulty communication between the brain and the gut microbiota (see Chapter 2).

Regarding specific diets, the low residue diet and the low FODMAP diet are two which appear in scientific literature most often. A low residue diet is about avoiding legumes, wholegrains, nuts, seeds and most fruits and vegetables. This is a restrictive diet which can't be safely followed for a long time but can be tried in periods of intense diarrhoea, nausea and pain. There is not much scientific evidence supporting its long-term use in IBD, though, and it requires vitamin and mineral supplementation.

The low FODMAP (fermentable oligosaccharides, disaccharides, monosaccharides and polyols) diet is receiving a lot of attention from researchers right now. FODMAPs are types of sugars which people with IBD often struggle to digest. Their large bowel then needs more water to process them and becomes distended, causing bowel symptoms such as bloating and pain. As I discussed in Chapter 1, quite a few IBD patients suffer from IBS symptoms on top of their IBD (i.e. bloating, pain, excessive wind) and the low FODMAP diet has been tested and found effective in reducing abdominal pain, bloating, wind and diarrhoea in IBS.[3, 4] In IBD, other than in those patients reporting ongoing bowel problems during remission, a low FODMAP diet may be useful in people with ostomies because it reduces excessive stool output and the frequency of emptying; however, importantly, it needs to be avoided by those with low stool output (where the risk of obstruction is increased as low FODMAP foods tend to make the stool output even lower).[5]

There are two steps to this diet:
1. restricting high FODMAP foods for six to eight weeks and in the meantime eating products low in FODMAPs;
2. slowly re-introducing high FODMAP products (one by one, to see how much you can tolerate).

You can find a list of high and low FODMAP foods elsewhere (see Self-help resources on page 132 for links to external websites), but briefly, examples of high FODMAP foods which need to be restricted are:

fruit (apples, apricots, mango, pears);

vegetables (cauliflower, garlic, onion, mushrooms, beans);

dairy (cow's milk, ice cream, hard cheeses, butter); and

legumes (lentils, chickpeas) and seeds (chia).

If fat absorption is a problem, a temporary restriction may be needed, but this should be supervised by a dietician or a doctor as fat is important to our health and cannot be avoided permanently.

Enteral nutrition (use of liquid food supplements or tube feeding) has good scientific evidence in some cases of IBD. It has a role in patients with CD, and particularly in children, where it can induce remission (see Chapter 4). It is less effective in adults.

In patients who have had an ileostomy, there is no specific diet recommended, though they are encouraged to drink plenty of fluids and choose foods rich in pectin (to thicken stool output), such as bananas, applesauce (stewed apple) or peanut butter.

Exercise

It is hard to dispute the value of physical activity. Next to healthy diet, it is the key to maintaining healthy weight and preventing obesity. Exercise extends our lives and also benefits mental health. But does it play any part in IBD?

After over 20 years of living with IBD, I have observed that during flares I exercise less. I am tired and a walk around the block is the maximum I can manage. But I have also noticed that my recovery from a flare is smoother when I exercise. I can reduce my pain by gentle stretching and I feel better when I walk in the sun. While flare-related fatigue takes weeks to subside, I get better more quickly if I go to the gym two to three times a week rather than resting all the time. It's a paradox, because exercise makes you tired but engaging in it also helps you fight fatigue.

Looking at the current state of research on physical activity and IBD, there is some evidence that exerice may help our immunity, strengthen muscles and bones, improve mood and reduce fatigue.[6] Yet, because very little research has examined the role of exercise in IBD, there are no IBD-specific guidelines on what is a good amount of physical activity for patients. We will have to wait a few years and in the meantime consult our doctors.

What we know about exercise and IBD, however, is that a big proportion of IBD patients are physically inactive and that people with IBD are less active than people without IBD. In a recent IBD survey, over 80% of respondents were categorised as either minimally active or inactive.[7] In terms of the types of physical activity IBD patients do, walking is the most common and running/jogging the most avoided.[7]

What reasons do IBD patients provide for not engaging in physical activity? Largely, this is due to abdominal or joint pain; fatigue; disease flare-up; increased toilet urgency and lack of toilet access.

It is a no-brainer that when IBD becomes active, physical activity decreases. We are simply too exhausted to continue our usual exercise routine. For example, in a recent study, 22% of people with mildly active CD reported being physically inactive versus 62% of people with severely-active CD.[7] At the same time, during flares, fatigue and mental problems become more common, and one of the important factors (other than disease activity) predicting low physical activity in IBD is depression.[7] It is thus important to seek help for mental disorders, not only because untreated they make you miserable and can result in suicide, but also because they prevent us from engaging in healthy practices such as exercise. This shows you yet another link between our physical and mental health, proving that there is no good health without mental health! My recommendation is thus to never forget about exercise. Speak to your doctor about what you can and cannot do and do as much as you are allowed.

Key points

- Diet and nutrition are important in IBD though there is currently no dietary regimen which can cure IBD.
- Many IBD patients, particularly children, are malnourished. Diet plays a supportive part in allowing those living with IBD to remain healthy and in reducing some of their IBD symptoms.
- Lactose sensitivity or intolerance is common in IBD. Saturated fats, sweeteners, chocolate, coffee and nuts are often reported as making the symptoms of IBD worse. Some vegetables such as beans, cabbage, broccoli, but also onion, may cause problems. Spicy food and whole grains may irritate the bowel.
- A visit to a dietician at some point during your IBD journey is highly recommended and can potentially improve your quality of life.
- A low-FODMAP diet may help some patients, especially those who have IBS in IBD and so suffer symptoms even during remission of their CD or UC.
- Exercise can help immunity, strengthen muscles and bones, improve mood and reduce fatigue.
- A big proportion of IBD patients are physically inactive. This is due to abdominal or joint pain; fatigue; disease flare-up; increased toilet urgency and lack of toilets. During flares, we tend to be less physically active than during remission.
- Coincidentally, fatigue and mental problems become more common when IBD is active, with one of the most important factors predicting low physical activity in IBD being depression.
- There are close links between physical activity, mood and fatigue. By scheduling regular physical activity, we can improve our mood and fatigue. Our IBD cannot be worse for it.

Chapter 12

Psychological treatments for IBD

Warsaw was covered with lilac blossom as I wandered through the cobbled streets of the Old Town. I wore a floral dress whose skirt danced around me in a gentle breeze. It was scorching hot, but I was oblivious to the clear blue sky and the inviting coolness of the old churches, my sole interest being to reach the nearby toilet. The road was littered with obstacles – crowds of absent-minded tourists, road works, areas of uneven surface, street merchants with stalls that took up nearly all available space. I was close to panic, for with each step I took, the loo appeared to be further away than before. But, this dream wasn't one of those in which you chase something and can't get to it. Overcoming the obstacles, I finally climbed a little hill on which the loo awaited – you might think a castle would make more sense at the top of the hill than a toilet, but you must have already guessed what my hierarchy of importance is! (By the way, no such place as this hill or loo exists in Warsaw's Old Town – it was purely a product of my imagination in the dream.)

The place was deserted. I felt thankful, as this was the type of loo that boasts a generous gap between the door and the floor – one of those where you can see the feet of someone inside. Don't you hate them? Who in their right mind would think of building a loo where you can hear even the faintest sound in the next-door cubicles? It wasn't someone with IBD, for sure.

Even today I recall the line of identical wooden doors and the untidy tiled floor. I got inside one of the cubicles and then something started to happen. A gurgling noise filled the space. I stared at the toilet in front of me as it burst with sewage. I opened the door to the next-door cubicle, and then to the next one, and the same happened there. All the toilets suddenly filled up with the yucky brown liquid, and not only filled but overflowed. Soon it was a poo flood. I tried to run but the wave of poo overtook me in the garden surrounding the loos. The last picture I have in my mind was of me drowning in a sea of human waste, disgusted but resigned.

This dream was so vivid that though I dreamt it over 20 years ago, I still remember the stench. I also recall my feelings: disgust, fear, panic, hopelessness and resignation. This was soon after I was diagnosed with IBD and this is how my sub-conscious mind had tried to come to terms with the disease.

Why am I telling you this? Psychotherapy (or talk therapy) is interested in our subconscious processes. People who struggle with a particular problem often dream about it, although it's not always obvious. Contemporary psychotherapy is not as crazy about dreams as the traditional psychoanalytical psychotherapy introduced by Sigmund Freud, an Austrian neurologist who believed dreams held the key to our inner struggles. But in my psychotherapy work, I have encountered some interesting dreams my patients have shared with me; I could learn from them on occasion what the patient couldn't put into words. Thus, if you dream interesting dreams, particularly if they repeat or bother you, and you undergo psychotherapy, don't ignore them but share them with your psychologist or psychiatrist. You may learn something valuable.

What is 'psychotherapy'? It is the overall term for the range of 'talking therapies' in which a variety of techniques and approaches can be used to help you deal with a problem. These include stress management, psychodynamic therapy, cognitive behaviour therapy (CBT), hypnotherapy, and acceptance commitment therapy (ACT) described below, but also many others. Its purpose is to facilitate change in your health and wellbeing. It's an evidence-based approach to treatment, meaning that it has been tested in a large number of studies which have shown it to work.[1] Of course, some therapies are more effective for a given problem than are others. The current guidelines for treatment in the UK (from the National Institute for Health and Care Excellence (NICE), see: www.nice.org.uk/guidance) recommend appropriate therapies for a variety of disorders, so if you are in any doubt about whether a type of psychotherapy you would like to try is evidence-based for your problem, you can check it there.

Similarly to what you read in Chapter 9 about antidepressants, while there is an evidence base for psychotherapy to be prescribed for anxiety and depression (or other mental symptoms or disorders) associated with IBD, studies have also examined whether it can improve bowel symptoms, disease course and pain in IBD patients.

The general conclusion has been that psychotherapy (of any type) is not recommended for all IBD patients – it is unlikely to harm you, but it may make no difference. It may, however, be useful in subgroups of patients who have unmet needs – for example, those with anxiety and/or depression in addition to their IBD ; those with IBD that is difficult to control or who suffer 'IBS in IBD'; younger patients; those recently diagnosed; or those who don't cope well with either an IBD diagnosis or some other aspect of the disease or treatment.[2-4] As such, psychotherapy is a supportive therapy in IBD but is not a treatment for IBD itself. There is currently little evidence that it has any impact on IBD activity in the long term, but anxiety, depression, pain and fatigue may improve as a result of psychotherapy.[5]

There are many types of psychotherapy and I will only focus on those most commonly used and tested with IBD patients.

Psychoeducation

Psychoeducation works through enhancing your knowledge of IBD and of associated psychological difficulties, but also explains what to expect as a patient, the role of health practitioners and the healthcare system. On its own, psychoeducation is not considered psychotherapy and is unlikely to work in IBD,[6] but many psychotherapies include elements of psychoeducation in their work and, in combination with evidence-based psychotherapies, it can be useful.

Stress management

Because stress is such an important issue in IBD (see Chapter 2), stress management has been considered a potential therapy in IBD. This type of therapy focuses on relaxation and stress reduction through some breathing exercises and problem-solving activities. Stress management may have some benefits for anxiety and IBD symptoms (including pain), but the evidence for this needs to be confirmed as studies to date are few and have conflicting results.[5, 7]

Psychodynamic therapy

Psychodynamic therapy is focused on helping you resolve problems with significant others in your life. In this therapy, you may be asked about your past life and delve into the past and present relationships. It's often a long-term therapy. Some studies report improvements in anxiety and depression, but there is little evidence of its usefulness for IBD symptoms or activity.[7]

CBT

CBT (cognitive-behavioural therapy) helps you modify your unhelpful thoughts and behaviours and improve your coping.

It's focused on the present rather than the past and provides you with new skills to deal with life's challenges. Courses of CBT are short-term, so may take weeks rather than months. It is presently one of the most widely used psychotherapies and the one which has been most extensively researched. It is the first line treatment for many mental disorders.

CBT appears to improve anxiety and depression in IBD, but there is presently no good evidence that it improves symptoms or the course of the disease.[4, 5, 7] It works best if it is applied to a single behaviour or symptom[8] so you may like to focus on one major problem, such as toilet dependence, during one course of CBT. And, it seems to be particularly useful for improving quality of life, anxiety, depression and coping in adolescents with IBD.[3]

Hypnotherapy

Hypnotherapy uses relaxation techniques and suggestions to improve health. It is a recognised medical technique and shouldn't be confused with the stage hypnosis you may have heard of on the media. Both may use similar techniques, but hypnotherapy should be carried out only by well-qualified health practitioners (i.e. doctors, nurses, psychologists) – in other words, the people from whom you would receive your other medical treatment. There are quite a lot of charlatans with minimum training around, so you should be careful who you visit, as hypnotherapy may have undesired effects in some patients, particularly those with a serious mental illness (see Chapter 13). These conditions should be addressed only by those who have appropriate training.

There is growing interest in hypnotherapy in IBD and also in other inflammatory illnesses.[8] A type of hypnotherapy called 'gut-directed hypnotherapy', which is focused on gastrointestinal functions, is a well-established treatment in other gastrointestinal conditions such as IBS.[9] According to the latest research, hypnotherapy may extend the period of remission in ulcerative colitis (UC) and reduce inflammation in the bowel.[8] No current data are available in Crohn's disease (CD). Many therapists successfully combine hypnotherapy with other treatments, such as CBT, so don't be surprised if you are offered it as part of your CBT treatment. It is usually a short-term therapy (5–7 sessions).

Other therapies

CBT may sometimes include an element of 'mindfulness', which is a form of meditation where you learn to be in the moment. It is then called 'mindfulness-based CBT'.

ACT (acceptance commitment therapy) is also sometimes combined with CBT – I personally use both these therapies together. ACT is focused on accepting the situation rather than changing our thoughts around it and can be useful (at least in my experience) in patients who don't like classic CBT.[10] ACT is often combined with mindfulness.

'Positive psychology' is another separate school of thought (as opposed to psychotherapy) which proposes many activities therapists may use with patients. If your therapist gives you some homework where you are asked to count your blessings and note them in a diary, it is a positive psychology activity. Positive psychology has one very important assumption which I use in daily life. It is around the concept of flow. Whenever we engage deeply in some activity – sport, art, handy work, meditation (or anything else which requires focus) – and are fully immersed in it to the point of losing self-consciousness (and thus we don't at the same time think about our marital problems or a nasty boss; we only live and breathe this activity), and enjoy the process, it is called a flow. You may improve your wellbeing by increasing the amount of time per day you engage in flow activities.

I am writing about it because for me flow is a sensation close to magic. No other psychological technique compares in terms of its immediate effect on my mood and I can use it relying solely on myself, as often as I like, and free of charge. If flow interests you, look for books by Mihaly Csíkszentmihaly.[11]

Key points

- Psychotherapy, or 'talking therapy', aims to facilitate a change in your health and wellbeing. It is not a solution for all people living with IBD. However, it is likely to help those with anxiety and/or depression; those with IBD that is difficult to control or who suffer from 'IBS in IBD'; younger patients; those recently diagnosed; or those who don't cope well either with an IBD diagnosis or with some other aspect of the disease or treatment. Talking therapy does not usually treat IBD, but it can help you manage it better and improve your quality of life.
- The most promising therapy to improve quality of life in IBD is CBT.
- Hypnotherapy undertaken by a qualified practitioner is a promising new treatment for symptoms of IBD, with some potential to extend remission in UC.
- To enhance your wellbeing, consider increasing the amount of time you spend in activities involving 'flow', a positive psychology concept where you are fully immersed in what you are doing – sport, art, handy work, meditation.

Chapter 13

Complementary and alternative therapies for IBD

In one of the many attempts to find a cure for my IBD, soon after my diagnosis my parents took me to a bio-energy therapist. Spiritual healers were in fashion in Poland at the time of my growing up. Most of the older people I knew watched a TV series where a Russian psychiatrist, Anatolij Kaszpirowski, healed with his voice. Hundreds of people in Eastern Europe were mesmerised by this healer and swore his sessions cured all possible ailments. My uncle, who had followed the series religiously, claimed Kaszpirowski's magnetic voice healed his varicose veins. All friends and neighbours knew someone whose eczema had disappeared, whose eyesight had miraculously improved or whose sexual prowess had never been as good as shortly after watching Kaszpirowski. Despite his initial success, Kaszpirowski's TV series ended abruptly, apparently because many of the viewers ended up in hospital with psychotic episodes. This is a possible side-effect of hypnosis when it is not done by a well-trained health professional. Hypnotherapy needs to be delivered face to face, or at least under close supervision, to ensure the risk of side-effects is minimised; Kaszpirowski used it via television, thus being far away from his patients and unable to supervise them.

While people believed in Kaszpirowski's powers, even in my teens I was reluctant to trust alternative medicine. The placebo effect (where the effect of a dummy drug or treatment is attributed to the patient's belief in its success rather than any active compound – in other words, faith works wonders) was something I read about early in my teens in a popular science book bought for me by my father. I was thus very sceptical when my parents suggested a visit to a bio-energy therapist. My parents themselves, both highly educated people, were reluctant about the whole idea of natural healing but when your child shrinks in front of your eyes and the standard medical treatment fails to help, you explore options you would otherwise sneer at.

The bio-energy therapist lived in a beautiful Art Deco villa on the outskirts of Warsaw and saw his patients in a greenhouse-like shed placed in one of the corners of the leafy garden. He healed with his touch. I was asked to lie down, and he then massaged my tummy while producing strange noises. The session took 20 minutes and throughout its whole duration I tried very hard to suppress my laughter. The wheezes, slurps and clicks of the tongue the man produced, the faces he made, and the tickling of the tummy were just a bit too much for my teen self. He ended his session by recommending that I wear malodourous sanitary pads for a week. My IBD was to be cured by the end of it. We never returned to this healer as my IBD was as bad a week later as it had always been.

My only other encounter with alternative medicine was through homeopathy. Through the recommendations of my aunt, our family doctor, who together with my parents spent hours thinking of how to cure the incurable, I was selected as an interesting 'case' by a group of Polish homeopaths. The interview with these people, mostly primary care doctors or doctors of other specialties who incorporated homeopathy in their practice, took a full day. By the end of it, they had explored and exhausted each minuscule aspect of my life, from the shape of my nipples (yes, they had a full scale of questions about them) to my emotional life and the personality of my first boyfriend. I then received several ampoules containing tiny candy-flavoured colourful balls, and sucked, chewed and swallowed them for quite some time. They differed from my therapy with the bio-energy therapist in that they had a strange effect. A few days after starting on them I developed my first cold sore. Obviously, I have no proof that the little sugary balls caused it. It could equally be that my body, weakened by chronic anaemia, opened itself to many different infections, but in my mind what homeopathy did for me was to give me a lip ulcer. Needless to say, there was no effect on my IBD. There has since been a significant amount of evidence questioning homeopathy's effectiveness in various chronic illnesses.[1]

What are CAMs?

It was many years before I took renewed interest in alternative IBD treatments. I had met some patients through my research and therapy work who used Chinese medicine, acupuncture or acupressure, some apparently with great results, but after my early experiences I had no faith or interest in these therapies. A couple of years ago, while editing a scientific book on IBD, my co-editor Dr Simon Knowles suggested that we should cover the topic and explore what science has to say about complementary and alternative medicine. I then learnt that there was quite a lot of research in the area. This discipline has even been acknowledged by the World Health Organization, who defined complementary and alternative medicine (CAM) as healthcare practices outside the prevailing healthcare system. CAMs include alternative practitioners such as homeopaths or healers; use of herbal medicine and dietary supplements; and self-care, including yoga or meditation but also prayer.

Do CAMs work?

While most healthcare systems do not pay for CAM therapies, and their efficacy is often questioned, many chronically ill people around the world use CAMs. Studies in IBD patients show that as many as 60% of them utilise CAMs. What people use varies between countries, with acupuncture being very popular among European IBD patients, for example. It is unsurprising to me that those who turn to CAMs usually report poorer health. If conventional medicine fails, as it did for me early in my disease, people explore non-conventional options. There are several studies showing that when conventional IBD therapy is successful, people are less likely to use CAMs.[2] Of interest are also the data showing that at least one third of IBD patients turning to CAMs are satisfied with this treatment. However, it is difficult to interpret studies on the relationship between use of CAMs and quality of life. Several of them show no effect, or even poorer quality of life in CAM users. This, however, may be because those with poor quality of life pursue CAMs more often than those whose IBD is well controlled. Therefore, their poorer quality of life may be a product of their IBD rather than the CAM treatment. It is hard to be certain.

We know CAMs are popular among IBD patients, but do they work? Looking at systematic reviews in relation to CAMs in IBD, there seems to be a lot of noise (so quite a number of studies) but no very clear message. Recent systematic reviews[3, 4] showed that acupuncture and herbal medicine have no effect on disease activity in IBD. This being said, there may be other CAM therapies not examined in these reviews that do have a role in IBD. For example, at present there are very few studies on yoga or meditation in IBD. Even with some encouraging preliminary results, we cannot yet be certain whether a large scale take-up of yoga or meditation would improve IBD activity.

As mental disorders, such as anxiety and depression, are

commonly associated with IBD, I looked at the evidence for the use of CAMs to improve mood at least, even if there was no evidence of improving bowel inflammation. With regard to depression, I found there was insufficient evidence to recommend the use of acupuncture,[5] and inconclusive data regarding the usefulness of yoga[6] or Chinese herbal medicine[7]; this means more studies are needed. I also looked at studies of CAMs in IBS, which, as I have said, often overlaps with IBD; this was to learn what effects CAMs can have on bowel pain or diarrhoea. I found no benefit with acupuncture,[8] but observed some benefits from yoga on bowel symptoms and associated anxiety[9] and of Chinese herbal medicine on diarrhoea and bowel pain.[10]

While we may need to wait a few years to get a definitive answer on the usefulness of CAMs in IBD, there is, however, one important finding from these studies now. They show that patients enjoy the holistic approach to care which is more common in CAM therapies than in standard treatment in IBD clinics. If we ask patients which type of care they prefer, many may choose CAMs because therapists have the time to speak and listen to them.

Key points

- CAMs include alternative therapies such as homeopathy; use of herbal medicine and dietary supplements; and self-care, including yoga, meditation and also prayer.
- As many as 60% of IBD patients utilise CAMs, and one third of these are satisfied with this treatment.
- Good studies in this area are limited but show that acupuncture and herbal medicine have no effect on disease activity in IBD. Other CAMs such as yoga and meditation have yet to be studied sufficiently.
- There are some encouraging preliminary findings for yoga for bowel symptoms and related anxiety, and for Chinese herbal medicine and diarrhoea and bowel pain, but again, more research is needed.
- People with IBD may, however, enjoy visiting CAM practitioners, even if the treatment's efficacy is doubtful, as these practitioners have the time to speak and listen to their patients.
- Hopefully in the future we can take what is useful about CAM therapies and adapt how standard IBD care is delivered to improve the patient experience.

Conclusion

I read last week in one of the most prestigious medical journals that the cure for Crohn's disease (CD) will have been found by 2032.[1] Though my mind tells me this is unlikely – there have been too many promising treatments over the years and, also, what about ulcerative colitis (UC)? – my heart leaps at the hope, for your sake and for mine. In the meantime, however, we need to learn to live with IBD and may as well try to tame it, given that 2032 is still a good few years away. My wish is that this book may help you on that journey. I decided to write it as I couldn't find a resource for patients which approached IBD care holistically and applied an integrated approach to understanding this complex illness.

I have tried to convey the current state of research on various topics relevant to living with IBD. I have also shared with you my experiences as a patient, and as a psychologist working with people suffering from IBD, in the hope that this knowledge may reassure you. I hope you have found some of what I have written useful and that your knowledge of IBD is now improved. IBD is an unusual illness, as disgusting as it is fascinating from the scientific point of view, but as with any problem in life, it can be managed (though we sometimes doubt it). Furthermore, improved understanding of what you are dealing with will help you on your path to living a healthier life. Finally, since a story which starts with a description of a perfect poo should have a matching finale, I wish you all clean and private loos which are always unoccupied and free to use.

There was a man from Cologne,

Who favoured pooping alone.

He built his own loo,

Soundproofing it through.

He since wolfs down bean calzone.

Self-help resources

Common blood tests used in IBD

Blood tests measure the presence of various substances in the blood. Here is a list of what your doctor is looking for, together with details of what are normal and abnormal readings.

- **CRP (C-reactive protein)**: Normal levels are below 3.0 mg/l. Above 3.0 mg/l indicates inflammation.
- **ESR (the erythrocyte sedimentation rate)**: Normal levels are 0–10 mm. Levels above 10 mm indicate inflammation.
- **Ferritin**: Normal levels are 15–165 μg/l. Levels below 15 μg/l indicate iron deficiency and anaemia.
- **Folic acid:** Normal levels in adults are 2–20 ng/ml, or 4.5–45.3 nmol/l. Normal levels in children are 5–21 ng/ml, or 11.3–47.6 nmol/l. Low levels of folic acid may indicate anaemia.
- **Haematocrit:** Normal levels for men are 45% to 52%; normal levels for women are 37% to 48%.
- **Haemoglobin**: Normal levels are 115–165 g/l. Levels below 115 g/l may indicate anaemia.
- **Iron**: Normal levels are 7–27 μmol/l. Levels below 7 may indicate anaemia.
- **Red cell count (RCC)**: Normal levels in men are 4.7 to 6.1 million cells/μl; normal levels in women are 4.2 to 5.4 million cells/μl. When the levels are lower than this it may indicate anaemia.

- **Vitamin B12**: Normal levels are 150–700 pmol/l.
- **Vitamin D:** Optimal levels are above 75 nmol/l.
- **White cell count (WCC)**: Normal levels are 4.0–11.0 x 109/l. Levels below 4.0 may indicate IBD is active.

If you would like to understand more about what is measured in blood tests, consider looking at Lab Tests Online which is a site sponsored by the Australian Government and dedicated to pathology testing: www.labtestsonline.org.au/

Dietary resources

- Low FODMAP diet: www.med.monash.edu/cecs/gastro/fodmap/description.html and
- http://shepherdworks.com.au/disease-information/low-fodmap-diet/#wrapper-wmw5541ba420746f
- FODMAP app: www.med.monash.edu/cecs/gastro/fodmap/iphone-app.html

Evidence-based resources

- NICE guidance – evidence-based guidelines on treating a variety of health conditions: www.nice.org.uk/guidance?unlid=
- Cochrane library – free summaries of systematic reviews on a variety of medical treatments and procedures: www.cochranelibrary.com/

Faecal incontinence and fistulas resource

- Managing bowel incontinence: http://s3-eu-west-1.amazonaws.com/files.crohnsandcolitis.org.uk/Publications/managing-bowel-incontinence-in-IBD.pdf
- If you would like to learn more about living with fistulas please see this resource published by Crohn's &

Colitis UK: http://s3-eu-west-1.amazonaws.com/files.
crohnsandcolitis.org.uk/Publications/fistula

IBD reports and guidelines

* An IBD in Australia report from 2013: www.
  crohnsandcolitis.com.au/research/studies-reports/
* RCP (Royal College of Physicians) 2017 IBD audit reporting
  on current state of affairs in IBD care in the UK and
  recommending changes for the future: www.rcplondon.
  ac.uk/projects/ibd-programme
* European Crohn's and Colitis Organisation (ECCO) – you
  will find European guidelines on IBD management here:
  www.ecco-ibd.eu/

Patient organisations

* Crohn's & Colitis UK: www.crohnsandcolitis.org.uk/
* Crohn's & Colitis Australia: www.crohnsandcolitis.com.au/
* Crohn's & Colitis Canada: www.crohnsandcolitis.ca/
* Crohn's & Colitis Foundation of America: www.ccfa.org
* The European Federation of Crohn's & Ulcerative Colitis
  Associations: www.efcca.org/

Parents' resources

* IBD in children: A parent's guide: www.crohnsandcolitis.
  org.uk/about-inflammatory-bowel-disease/publications/
  ibd-in-children-a-parents-guide
* Moving to adult care: http://s3-eu-west-1.amazonaws.
  com/files.crohnsandcolitis.org.uk/Publications/transition-
  moving-to-adult-IBD-care
* Children with IBD: guide for schools: http://s3-eu-
  west-1.amazonaws.com/files.crohnsandcolitis.org.uk/
  Publications/children-schools-IBD-guide.pdf

- Talking to children about parents' IBD: http://s3-eu-west-1.amazonaws.com/files.crohnsandcolitis.org.uk/Publications/talking-to-my-child-about-my-IBD.pdf

Psychological resources for those living with IBD

- Self-directed psychotherapy (CBT) for IBD: www.tameyourgut.com
- Self-directed psychotherapy (CBT) for IBD: www.ibdclinic.org.au/

Resources for students with IBD

- A guide for students: http://s3-eu-west-1.amazonaws.com/files.crohnsandcolitis.org.uk/Publications/students-with-IBD-students.pdf

Other resources

- North American Society for Pediatric Gastroenterology, Hepatology and Nutrition: NASPGHAN.org
- Mayo Clinic: MayoClinic.org/ibd/

Toilet locator apps

- Toilocator – www.toilocator.com – a crowdsourced app for finding a public toilet or bathroom or restroom around the world.
- Bathroom Scout – https://bathroom-scout.en.aptoide.com/ – allows you easily to find about 1,800,000 bathrooms and restrooms worldwide. This includes public toilets as well as restrooms in restaurants and other facilities.
- Flush Toilet Finder – www.jrustonapps.com/apps/flush-toilet-finder – 100,000 public loos all around the world showing which have disabled access, a fee for usage or require a key
- Australian public toilet map: https://toiletmap.gov.au/Find

References

Preface

1. Wikipedia. Bristol Stool Scale. https://en.wikipedia.org/wiki/Bristol_stool_scale (accessed 7 March 2018).
2. Knowles SR, Mikocka-Walus AA (eds). *Psychological Aspects of Inflammatory Bowel Disease: A Biopsychosocial Approach.* London: Routledge; 2015.

Chapter 1

1. Mulder DJ, Noble AJ, Justinich CJ, Duffin JM. A tale of two diseases: the history of inflammatory bowel disease. *Journal of Crohn's & Colitis* 2014;8(5):341–8.
2. Wilks S. The morbid appearance of the intestine of Miss Banks. *Medical Times and Gazette* 1859;2:264.
3. Zhang YZ, Li YY. Inflammatory bowel disease: pathogenesis. *World Journal of Gastroenterology* 2014;20(1):91–9.
4. Katakura K, Watanabe H, Ohira H. Innate immunity and inflammatory bowel disease: a review of clinical evidence and future application. *Clinical Journal of Gastroenterology* 2013;6(6):415–9.
5. Koloski NA, Bret L, Radford-Smith G. Hygiene hypothesis in inflammatory bowel disease: a critical review of the literature. *World Journal of Gastroenterology* 2008;14(2):165–73.
6. Molodecky NA, Kaplan GG. Environmental risk factors for inflammatory bowel disease. *Gastroenterology & Hepatology* 2010;6(5):339–46.

7. Bernstein CN, Shanahan F. Disorders of a modern lifestyle: reconciling the epidemiology of inflammatory bowel diseases. *Gut* 2008;57(9):1185–91.

8. Sakamoto N, Kono S, Wakai K, Fukuda Y, Satomi M, Shimoyama T, et al. Dietary risk factors for inflammatory bowel disease: a multicenter case-control study in Japan. *Inflammatory Bowel Diseases* 2005;11(2):154–63.

9. Amre DK, D'Souza S, Morgan K, Seidman G, Lambrette P, Grimard G, et al. Imbalances in dietary consumption of fatty acids, vegetables, and fruits are associated with risk for Crohn's disease in children. *The American Journal of Gastroenterology* 2007;102(9):2016–25.

10. Asthana AK, Gibson PR. IBS in IBD and psychological implications. In: Knowles SR, Mikocka-Walus A (eds). *Psychological Aspects of Inflammatory Bowel Disease: A Biopsychosocial Approach.* London: Routledge; 2015. p. 84–92.

11. Aguas M, Garrigues V, Bastida G, Nos P, Ortiz V, Fernandez A, et al. Prevalence of irritable bowel syndrome (IBS) in first-degree relatives of patients with inflammatory bowel disease (IBD). *Journal of Crohn's & Colitis* 2011;5(3):227–33.

11A. Koloski NA, Jones M, Talley NJ. Evidence that independent gut-to-brain and brain-to-gut pathways operate in the irritable bowel syndrome and functional dyspepsia: a one-year population-based prospective study. *Aliment Pharmacol Ther* 2016; 44: 592–600. DOI:10.1111/apt.13738

12. Price JR, Mitchell E, Tidy E, Hunot V. Cognitive behaviour therapy for chronic fatigue syndrome in adults. *The Cochrane Database of Systematic Reviews* 2008(3):CD001027.

13. Lakatos PL, Lakatos L. Risk for colorectal cancer in ulcerative colitis: changes, causes and management strategies. *World Journal of Gastroenterology* 2008;14(25):3937–47.

14. Jess T, Rungoe C, Peyrin-Biroulet L. Risk of colorectal cancer in patients with ulcerative colitis: a meta-analysis of population-based cohort studies. *Clinical Gastroenterology and Hepatology: The Official Clinical Practice Journal of the American Gastroenterological Association* 2012;10(6):639–45.

15. Basseri RJ, Basseri B, Vassilaki ME, Melmed GY, Ippoliti A, Vasiliauskas EA, et al. Colorectal cancer screening and

surveillance in Crohn's colitis. *Journal of Crohn's & Colitis* 2012;6(8):824–9.

16. Knowles SR, Macrae FA. IBD, cancer, and its psychological impact. In: Knowles SR, Mikocka-Walus A (eds). *Psychological Aspects of Inflammatory Bowel Disease: A Biopsychosocial Approach*. London: Routledge; 2014. pp. 93–101.

17. Mason M, Siegel CA. Do inflammatory bowel disease therapies cause cancer? *Inflammatory Bowel Diseases* 2013;19(6):1306–21.

18. Bernstein CN, Nugent Z, Targownik LE, Singh H, Lix LM. Predictors and risks for death in a population-based study of persons with IBD in Manitoba. *Gut* 2015;64(9):1403–11.

19. Caini S, Bagnoli S, Palli D, Saieva C, Ceroti M, Bendinelli B, et al. Total and cancer mortality in a cohort of ulcerative colitis and Crohn's disease patients: The Florence inflammatory bowel disease study, 1978–2010. *Digestive and Liver Disease Journal* 2016;48(10):1162–7.

20. Canavan C, Abrams KR, Mayberry JF. Meta-analysis: mortality in Crohn's disease. *Alimentary Pharmacology & Therapeutics* 2007;25(8):861–70.

21. Hoivik ML, Moum B, Solberg IC, Henriksen M, Cvancarova M, Bernklev T, et al. Work disability in inflammatory bowel disease patients 10 years after disease onset: results from the IBSEN Study. *Gut* 2013;62(3):368–75.

22. Bernklev T, Jahnsen J, Lygren I, Henriksen M, Vatn M, Moum B. Health-related quality of life in patients with inflammatory bowel disease measured with the short form-36: psychometric assessments and a comparison with general population norms. *Inflammatory Bowel Diseases* 2005;11(10):909–18.

23. CCA. The economic costs of Crohn's disease and ulcerative colitis. *Melbourne: Crohn's and Colitis of Australia* 2007.

24. Boonen A, Dagnelie PC, Feleus A, Hesselink MA, Muris JW, Stockbrugger RW, et al. The impact of inflammatory bowel disease on labor force participation: results of a population sampled case-control study. *Inflammatory bowel diseases.* 2002;8(6):382–9.

25. The IBD Standards Group. Standards for the Healthcare of People who have Inflammatory Bowel Disease (IBD): 2013 update 2013 [Available from: http://www.ibdstandards.org.uk/uploaded_files/IBDstandards.pdf.]

26. Burisch J, Jess T, Martinato M, Lakatos PL, EpiCom E. The burden of inflammatory bowel disease in Europe. *Journal of Crohn's & colitis*. 2013;7(4):322–37.

Chapter 2

1. Sokol H, Pigneur B, Watterlot L, Lakhdari O, Bermudez-Humaran LG, Gratadoux JJ, et al. Faecalibacterium prausnitzii is an anti-inflammatory commensal bacterium identified by gut microbiota analysis of Crohn disease patients. *Proceedings of the National Academy of Sciences of the United States of America* 2008;105(43):16731–6.

2. Sartor RB. Therapeutic manipulation of the enteric microflora in inflammatory bowel diseases: antibiotics, probiotics, and prebiotics. *Gastroenterology* 2004;126(6):1620–33.

3. Anderson JL, Edney RJ, Whelan K. Systematic review: faecal microbiota transplantation in the management of inflammatory bowel disease. *Alimentary Pharmacology & Therapeutics* 2012;36(6):503–16.

4. David LA, Maurice CF, Carmody RN, Gootenberg DB, Button JE, Wolfe BE, et al. Diet rapidly and reproducibly alters the human gut microbiome. *Nature* 2014;505(7484):559–63.

5. Critch J, Day AS, Otley A, King-Moore C, Teitelbaum JE, Shashidhar H, et al. Use of enteral nutrition for the control of intestinal inflammation in pediatric Crohn disease. *Journal of Pediatric Gastroenterology and Nutrition* 2012;54(2):298–305.

6. Collins SM, Bercik P. The relationship between intestinal microbiota and the central nervous system in normal gastrointestinal function and disease. *Gastroenterology* 2009;136(6):2003–14.

7. Bested AC, Logan AC, Selhub EM. Intestinal microbiota, probiotics and mental health: from Metchnikoff to modern advances: Part I – autointoxication revisited. *Gut Pathogens* 2013;5(1):5.

8. Bonaz BL, Bernstein CN. Brain–gut interactions in inflammatory bowel disease. *Gastroenterology* 2013;144(1):36–49.

9. Agostini A, Filippini N, Cevolani D, Agati R, Leoni C, Tambasco R, et al. Brain functional changes in patients with

ulcerative colitis: a functional magnetic resonance imaging study on emotional processing. *Inflammatory Bowel Diseases* 2011;17(8):1769–77.

10. Mayer EA, Bradesi S, Gupta A, Katibian DJ. The brain–gut axis and psychological processes in IBD. In: Knowles SR, Mikocka-Walus A (eds). *Psychological Aspects of Inflammatory Bowel Disease: A Biopsychosocial Approach.* London: Routledge; 2015. pp. 20–9.

11. Mayer EA. *The Mind–Gut Connection: How the Hidden Conversation Within Our Bodies Impacts Our Mood, Our Choices, and Our Overall Health:* HarperWave; 2016.

12. Sexton KA, Bernstein CN. Stress, distress and IBD. In: Knowles SR, Mikocka-Walus A (eds). *Psychological Aspects of Inflammatory Bowel Disease: A Biopsychosocial Approach.* London: Routledge; 2015. pp. 10–9.

13. Targownik LE, Sexton KA, Bernstein MT, Beatie B, Sargent M, Walker JR, et al. The Relationship Among Perceived Stress, Symptoms, and Inflammation in Persons With Inflammatory Bowel Disease. *The American Journal of Gastroenterology* 2015;110(7):1001–12; quiz 13.

14. Mikocka-Walus A, Knowles SR, Keefer L, Graff L. Controversies revisited: a systematic review of the comorbidity of depression and anxiety with inflammatory bowel diseases. *Inflammatory Bowel Diseases* 2016;22(3):752–62.

15. Mikocka-Walus A, Pittet V, Rossel JB, von Kanel R, Swiss IBDCSG. Symptoms of depression and anxiety are independently associated with clinical recurrence of inflammatory bowel disease. *Clinical Gastroenterology and Hepatology: The Official Clinical Practice Journal of the American Gastroenterological Association* 2016;14(6):829–35 e1.

Chapter 3

1. van der Have M, van der Aalst KS, Kaptein AA, Leenders M, Siersema PD, Oldenburg B, et al. Determinants of health-related quality of life in Crohn's disease: a systematic review and meta-analysis. *Journal of Crohn's & Colitis* 2014;8(2):93–106.

2. Keeton RL, Mikocka-Walus A, Andrews JM. Concerns and worries in people living with inflammatory bowel disease

(IBD): A mixed methods study. *Journal of Psychosomatic Research* 2015;78(6):573–8.

3. Sexton KA, Bernstein CN. Stress, distress and IBD. In: Knowles SR, Mikocka-Walus A (eds). *Psychological Aspects of Inflammatory Bowel Disease: A Biopsychosocial approach.* London: Routledge; 2015. pp. 10–9.

4. Taylor S. Health Psychology. New York, US: McGraw-Hill; 2018.

5. McCombie AM, Mulder RT, Gearry RB. How IBD patients cope with IBD: a systematic review. *Journal of Crohn's & Colitis* 2013;7(2):89–106.

6. Holt-Lunstad J, Smith TB, Baker M, Harris T, Stephenson D. Loneliness and social isolation as risk factors for mortality: a meta-analytic review. *Perspectives on Psychological Science: A Journal of the Association for Psychological Science* 2015;10(2):227–37.

7. Camara RJ, Lukas PS, Begre S, Pittet V, von Kanel R, Swiss Inflammatory Bowel Disease Cohort Study G. Effects of social support on the clinical course of Crohn's disease. *Inflammatory Bowel Diseases* 2011;17(6):1277–86.

8. Malik S, Coulson NS. The therapeutic potential of the internet: exploring self-help processes in an internet forum for young people with inflammatory bowel disease. *Gastroenterology Nursing: The Official Journal of the Society of Gastroenterology Nurses and Associates* 2011;34(6):439–48.

9. Jordan C, Sin J, Fear NT, Chalder T. A systematic review of the psychological correlates of adjustment outcomes in adults with inflammatory bowel disease. *Clinical Psychology Review* 2016;47:28–40.

Chapter 4

1. Benchimol EI, Fortinsky KJ, Gozdyra P, Van den Heuvel M, Van Limbergen J, Griffiths AM. Epidemiology of pediatric inflammatory bowel disease: a systematic review of international trends. *Inflammatory Bowel Diseases* 2011;17(1):423–39.

2. Zachos M, Tondeur M, Griffiths AM. Enteral nutritional therapy for induction of remission in Crohn's disease. *The Cochrane Database of Systematic Reviews* 2007(1):CD000542.

3. Szigethy E, Craig AE, Iobst EA, Grand RJ, Keljo D, DeMaso D, et

al. Profile of depression in adolescents with inflammatory bowel disease: implications for treatment. *Inflammatory Bowel Diseases* 2009;15(1):69–74.

4. Greenley RN, Hommel KA, Nebel J, Raboin T, Li SH, Simpson P, et al. A meta-analytic review of the psychosocial adjustment of youth with inflammatory bowel disease. *Journal of Pediatric Psychology* 2010;35(8):857–69.

Chapter 5

1. Trachter AB, Rogers AI, Leiblum SR. Inflammatory bowel disease in women: impact on relationship and sexual health. *Inflammatory Bowel Diseases* 2002;8(6):413–21.

2. Davies RJ, O'Connor BI, Victor C, MacRae HM, Cohen Z, McLeod RS. A prospective evaluation of sexual function and quality of life after ileal pouch-anal anastomosis. *Diseases of the Colon and Rectum* 2008;51(7):1032–5.

3. Timmer A, Bauer A, Dignass A, Rogler G. Sexual function in persons with inflammatory bowel disease: a survey with matched controls. *Clinical Gastroenterology and Hepatology: The Official Clinical Practice Journal of the American Gastroenterological Association* 2007;5(1):87–94.

4. Timmer A, Bauer A, Kemptner D, Furst A, Rogler G. Determinants of male sexual function in inflammatory bowel disease: a survey-based cross-sectional analysis in 280 men. *Inflammatory Bowel Diseases* 2007;13(10):1236–43.

5. Moody G, Probert CS, Srivastava EM, Rhodes J, Mayberry JF. Sexual dysfunction amongst women with Crohn's disease: a hidden problem. *Digestion* 1992;52(3–4):179–83.

6. Cornish JA, Tan E, Simillis C, Clark SK, Teare J, Tekkis PP. The risk of oral contraceptives in the etiology of inflammatory bowel disease: a meta-analysis. *The American Journal of Gastroenterology* 2008;103(9):2394–400.

7. Zapata LB, Paulen ME, Cansino C, Marchbanks PA, Curtis KM. Contraceptive use among women with inflammatory bowel disease: A systematic review. *Contraception* 2010;82(1):72–85.

8. Nguyen GC, Sam J. Rising prevalence of venous thromboembolism and its impact on mortality among

hospitalized inflammatory bowel disease patients. *The American Journal of Gastroenterology* 2008;103(9):2272–80.

9.   WHO. *Improving Access to Quality Care in Family Planning: Medical Eligibility Criteria for Contraceptive Use*. Geneva: World Health Organization. Dept. of Reproductive Health and Research; 2000.

10. RCOG. *Male and Female Sterilisation* (Evidence-based Clinical Guideline No. 4). London: RCOG Press; 2004.

11. Mountifield R. Sexual function, contraception and IBD. In: Knowles SR, Mikocka-Walus A (eds). *Psychological Aspects of Inflammatory Bowel Disease: A Biopsychosocial Approach*. London: Routledge; 2015. pp. 65–73.

12. Abhyankar A, Ham M, Moss AC. Meta-analysis: the impact of disease activity at conception on disease activity during pregnancy in patients with inflammatory bowel disease. *Alimentary Pharmacology & Therapeutics* 2013;38(5):460–6.

13. Rajaratnam SG, Eglinton TW, Hider P, Fearnhead NS. Impact of ileal pouch-anal anastomosis on female fertility: meta-analysis and systematic review. *International Journal of Colorectal Disease* 2011;26(11):1365–74.

14. Orholm M, Munkholm P, Langholz E, Nielsen OH, Sorensen TI, Binder V. Familial occurrence of inflammatory bowel disease. *The New England Journal of Medicine* 1991;324(2):84–8.

15. Bennett RA, Rubin PH, Present DH. Frequency of inflammatory bowel disease in offspring of couples both presenting with inflammatory bowel disease. *Gastroenterology* 1991;100(6):1638–43.

16. van der Woude CJ, Ardizzone S, Bengtson MB, Fiorino G, Fraser G, Katsanos K, et al. The second European evidenced-based consensus on reproduction and pregnancy in inflammatory bowel disease. *Journal of Crohn's & Colitis* 2015;9(2):107–24.

17. Casanova MJ, Chaparro M, Domenech E, Barreiro-de Acosta M, Bermejo F, Iglesias E, et al. Safety of thiopurines and anti-TNF-alpha drugs during pregnancy in patients with inflammatory bowel disease. *The American Journal of Gastroenterology* 2013;108(3):433–40.

18. Kozlowski RD, Steinbrunner JV, MacKenzie AH, Clough JD, Wilke WS, Segal AM. Outcome of first-trimester exposure to low-dose methotrexate in eight patients with rheumatic disease. *American Journal of Medicine* 1990;88(6):589–92.

19. Viktil KK, Engeland A, Furu K. Outcomes after anti-rheumatic drug use before and during pregnancy: a cohort study among 150,000 pregnant women and expectant fathers. *Scandinavian Journal of Rheumatology* 2012;41(3):196–201.
20. Park-Wyllie L, Mazzotta P, Pastuszak A, Moretti ME, Beique L, Hunnisett L, et al. Birth defects after maternal exposure to corticosteroids: prospective cohort study and meta-analysis of epidemiological studies. *Teratology* 2000;62(6):385–92.
21. Cornish J, Tan E, Teare J, Teoh TG, Rai R, Clark SK, et al. A meta-analysis on the influence of inflammatory bowel disease on pregnancy. *Gut* 2007;56(6):830–7.

Chapter 6

1. Piront P, Louis E, Latour P, Plomteux O, Belaiche J. Epidemiology of inflammatory bowel diseases in the elderly in the province of Liege. *Gastroenterology Clinical Biology* 2002;26(2):157–61.
2. Takeuchi K, Smale S, Premchand P, Maiden L, Sherwood R, Thjodleifsson B, et al. Prevalence and mechanism of nonsteroidal anti-inflammatory drug-induced clinical relapse in patients with inflammatory bowel disease. *Clinical Gastroenterology and Hepatology: The Official Clinical PracticeJjournal of the American Gastroenterological Association* 2006;4(2):196–202.
3. Cottone M, Kohn A, Daperno M, Armuzzi A, Guidi L, D'Inca R, et al. Advanced age is an independent risk factor for severe infections and mortality in patients given anti-tumor necrosis factor therapy for inflammatory bowel disease. *Clinical Gastroenterology and Hepatology: The Official Clinical Practice Journal of the American Gastroenterological Association* 2011;9(1):30–5.

Chapter 7

1. Boyapati R, Leung C. Cross-cultural aspects of IBD. In: Knowles SR, Mikocka-Walus A (eds). *Psychological Aspects of Inflammatory Bowel Disease: A Biopsychosocial Approach.* London: Routledge; 2015. pp. 140–9.
2. Dimsdale JE. Stalked by the past: the influence of ethnicity on health. *Psychosometric Medicine* 2000;62(2):161–70.

3. Walker DG, Williams HR, Kane SP, Mawdsley JE, Arnold J, McNeil I, et al. Differences in inflammatory bowel disease phenotype between South Asians and Northern Europeans living in North West London, UK. *The American Journal of Gastroenterology* 2011;106(7):1281–9.

4. Hou JK, El-Serag H, Thirumurthi S. Distribution and manifestations of inflammatory bowel disease in Asians, Hispanics, and African Americans: a systematic review. *The American Journal of Gastroenterology* 2009;104(8):2100–9.

5. Levenstein S, Li Z, Almer S, Barbosa A, Marquis P, Moser G, et al. Cross-cultural variation in disease-related concerns among patients with inflammatory bowel disease. *The American Journal of Gastroenterology* 2001;96(6):1822–30.

6. Finlay DG, Basu D, Sellin JH. Effect of race and ethnicity on perceptions of inflammatory bowel disease. *Inflammatory Bowel Diseases* 2006;12(6):503–7.

7. Dabadie A, Troadec F, Heresbach D, Siproudhis L, Pagenault M, Bretagne JF. Transition of patients with inflammatory bowel disease from pediatric to adult care. *Gastroenterology Clinical Biology* 2008;32(5 Pt 1):451–9.

8. Knowles SR. Future directions in IBD: eHealth. In: Knowles SR, Mikocka-Walus A (eds). *Psychological Aspects of Inflammatory Bowel Disease: A Biopsychosocial Approach.* London: Routledge; 2014. pp. 207–15.

9. Fortinsky KJ, Fournier MR, Benchimol EI. Internet and electronic resources for inflammatory bowel disease: a primer for providers and patients. *Inflammatory Bowel Disease* 2012;18(6):1156–63.

10. Knowles SR, Mikocka-Walus A. Utilization and efficacy of internet-based eHealth technology in gastroenterology: a systematic review. *Scandinavian Journal of Gastroenterology* 2014;49(4):387–408.

11. Sack C, Phan VA, Grafton R, Holtmann G, van Langenberg DR, Brett K. A chronic care model significantly decreases costs and healthcare utilisation in patients with inflammatory bowel disease. *Journal of Crohn's & Colitis* 2012;6(3):302–10.

12. Mikocka-Walus A, Andrews JM, Rampton D, Goodhand J, van der Woude J, Bernstein CN. How can we improve models of care in inflammatory bowel disease? An international survey of IBD

health professionals. *Journal of Crohn's & Colitis* 2014;8(12):1668–74.

13. Mikocka-Walus A, Power M, Rook L, Robins G. CCUK York Walk Planning Committee. What Do Participants of the Crohn's and Colitis UK (CCUK) Annual York Walk Think of Their Inflammatory Bowel Disease Care? A Short Report on a Survey. *Gastroenterology Nursing: The Official Journal of the Society of Gastroenterology Nurses and Associates* 2016. 41(1), 59–64.

Chapter 8

1. Mikocka-Walus AA, Moulds LG, Rollbusch N, Andrews JM. 'It's a tube up your bottom; it makes people nervous': the experience of anxiety in initial colonoscopy patients. *Gastroenterology Nursing: The Official Journal of the Society of Gastroenterology Nurses and Associates* 2012;35(6):392–401.

2. Bessissow T, Van Keerberghen CA, Van Oudenhove L, Ferrante M, Vermeire S, Rutgeerts P, et al. Anxiety is associated with impaired tolerance of colonoscopy preparation in inflammatory bowel disease and controls. *Journal of Crohn's & Colitis* 2013;7(11):e580–7.

3. Bechtold ML, Puli SR, Othman MO, Bartalos CR, Marshall JB, Roy PK. Effect of music on patients undergoing colonoscopy: a meta-analysis of randomized controlled trials. *Digestive Diseases and Sciences* 2009;54(1):19–24.

Chapter 9

1. Mountifield R, Andrews JM, Mikocka-Walus A, Bampton P. Covert dose reduction is a distinct type of medication non-adherence observed across all care settings in inflammatory bowel disease. *Journal of Crohn's & Colitis* 2014;8(12):1723–9.

2. Hendy P, Inspector Y, Hart A. Standard medical care, side effects and compliance. In: Knowles SR, Mikocka-Walus A (eds). *Psychological Aspects of Inflammatory Bowel Disease: A Biopsychosocial Approach.* London: Routledge; 2015.

3. Ford AC, Quigley EM, Lacy BE, Lembo AJ, Saito YA, Schiller LR, et al. Effect of antidepressants and psychological therapies, including hypnotherapy, in irritable bowel syndrome: systematic

review and meta-analysis. *The American Journal of Gastroenterology* 2014;109(9):1350–65; quiz 66.

4. Ford AC, Talley NJ, Schoenfeld PS, Quigley EM, Moayyedi P. Efficacy of antidepressants and psychological therapies in irritable bowel syndrome: systematic review and meta-analysis. *Gut* 2009;58(3):367–78.

5. Grover M, Drossman DA. Psychotropic agents in functional gastrointestinal disorders. *Current Opinion in Pharmacology* 2008;8(6):715–23.

6. Kirsch I. *The Emperor's New Drugs: Exploding the Antidepressant Myth.* New York: Basic Books; 2009.

7. Rayner L, Price A, Evans A, Valsraj K, Higginson IJ, Hotopf M. Antidepressants for depression in physically ill people. *The Cochrane Database of Systematic Reviews* 2010(3):CD007503.

8. Haapamaki J, Tanskanen A, Roine RP, Blom M, Turunen U, Mantyla J, et al. Medication use among inflammatory bowel disease patients: excessive consumption of antidepressants and analgesics. *Scandinavian Journal of Gastroenterology* 2013;48(1):42–50.

9. Fuller-Thomson E, Sulman J. Depression and inflammatory bowel disease: findings from two nationally representative Canadian surveys. *Inflammatory Bowel Diseases* 2006;12(8):697–707.

10. Mikocka-Walus AA, Turnbull DA, Moulding NT, Wilson IG, Andrews JM, Holtmann GJ. Antidepressants and inflammatory bowel disease: a systematic review. *Clinical Practice and Epidemiology in Mental Health* 2006;2:24.

11. Mikocka-Walus A, Clarke D, Gibson P. Can antidepressants influence the course of inflammatory bowel disease? The current state of research. *European Gastroenterology & Hepatology* 2009;5:48–53.

12. Macer B, Prady S, Mikocka-Walus A. Antidepressants in Inflammatory Bowel Disease: A systematic review. *Inflammatory bowel diseases.* 2017; 23(4):534–550.

Chapter 10

1. Ananthakrishnan AN, Gainer VS, Cai T, Perez RG, Cheng SC, Savova G, et al. Similar risk of depression and anxiety following surgery or hospitalization for Crohn's disease and ulcerative

colitis. *The American Journal of Gastroenterology* 2013;108(4):594–601.

2. Frolkis AD, Dykeman J, Negron ME, Debruyn J, Jette N, Fiest KM, et al. Risk of surgery for inflammatory bowel diseases has decreased over time: a systematic review and meta-analysis of population-based studies. *Gastroenterology* 2013;145(5):996–1006.

3. Lewis RT, Maron DJ. Efficacy and complications of surgery for Crohn's disease. *Gastroenterology & Hepatology* 2010;6(9):587–96.

4. Hwang JM, Varma MG. Surgery for inflammatory bowel disease. *World Journal of Gastroenterology* 2008;14(17):2678–90.

5. Blondel-Kucharski F, Chircop C, Marquis P, Cortot A, Baron F, Gendre JP, et al. Health-related quality of life in Crohn's disease: a prospective longitudinal study in 231 patients. *The American Journal of Gastroenterology* 2001;96(10):2915–20.

6. Ko CY, Rusin LC, Schoetz DJ, Jr., Moreau L, Coller JC, Murray JJ, et al. Long-term outcomes of the ileal pouch anal anastomosis: the association of bowel function and quality of life 5 years after surgery. *Journal of Surgical Research* 2001;98(2):102–7.

7. Spinelli A, Pagnini F. Patients and IBD surgery: Rightful fears and preconceptions. In: Knowles SR, Mikocka-Walus A (eds). *Psychological Aspects of Inflammatory Bowel Disease: A Biopsychosocial Approach.* London: Routledge; 2014.

8. Silva MA, Ratnayake G, Deen KI. Quality of life of stoma patients: temporary ileostomy versus colostomy. *World Journal of Surgery* 2003;27(4):421–4.

9. El-Tawil A, Nightingale P. Living with stoma: long-term effects on patients' quality of life. *Journal of Clinical Cell Immunology* 2013;4(145):2.

10. Bennis M, Tiret E. Surgical management of ulcerative colitis. *Langenbeck's Archives of Surgery* 2012;397(1):11–7.

Chapter 11

1. Hartman C, Eliakim R, Shamir R. Nutritional status and nutritional therapy in inflammatory bowel diseases. *World Journal of Gastroenterology* 2009;15(21):2570–8.

2. Haller D, Antoine JM, Bengmark S, Enck P, Rijkers GT, Lenoir-Wijnkoop I. Guidance for substantiating the evidence for beneficial effects of probiotics: probiotics in chronic inflammatory

bowel disease and the functional disorder irritable bowel syndrome. *Journal of Nutrition* 2010;140(3):690S–7S.

3.   Charlebois A, Rosenfeld G, Bressler B. The impact of dietary interventions on the symptoms of inflammatory bowel disease: a systematic review. *Critical Review of Food Science and Nutrition* 2016;56(8):1370–8.

4.   Marsh A, Eslick EM, Eslick GD. Does a diet low in FODMAPs reduce symptoms associated with functional gastrointestinal disorders? A comprehensive systematic review and meta-analysis. *European Journal of Nutrition* 2016;55(3):897–906.

5.   Shepherd SJ. Diet, nutrition and mental health in IBD. In: Knowles SR, Mikocka-Walus A (eds). *Psychological Aspects of Inflammatory Bowel Disease: A Biopsychosocial Approach*. London: Routledge; 2014. pp. 118–29.

6.   Bilski J, Mazur-Bialy A, Brzozowski B, Magierowski M, Zahradnik-Bilska J, Wójcik D, et al. Can exercise affect the course of inflammatory bowel disease? Experimental and clinical evidence. *Pharmacology Report* 2016;68(4):827–36.

7.   Tew GA, Jones K, Mikocka-Walus A. Physical activity habits, limitations and predictors in people with inflammatory bowel disease: a large cross-sectional online survey. *Inflammatory Bowel Diseases* 2016; 22(12): 2933–2942.

Chapter 12

1.   Roth A, Fonagy P. *What Works for Whom? A Critical Review of Psychotherapy Research*. 2nd ed. New York: Guilford Press; 2005.

2.   Miehsler W, Weichselberger M, Offerlbauer-Ernst A, Dejaco C, Reinisch W, Vogelsang H, et al. Which patients with IBD need psychological interventions? A controlled study. *Inflammatory bowel Diseases* 2008;14(9):1273–80.

3.   Timmer A, Preiss JC, Motschall E, Rucker G, Jantschek G, Moser G. Psychological interventions for treatment of inflammatory bowel disease. *The Cochrane Database of Systematic Reviews* 2011(2):CD006913.

4.   Mikocka-Walus A, Bampton P, Hetzel D, Hughes P, Esterman A, Andrews JM. Cognitive-behavioural therapy has no effect

on disease activity but improves quality of life in subgroups of patients with inflammatory bowel disease: a pilot randomised controlled trial. *BMC Gastroenterology* 2015;15:54.

5. McCombie AM, Mulder RT, Gearry RB. Psychotherapy for inflammatory bowel disease: a review and update. *Journal of Crohn's & Colitis* 2013;7(12):935–49.

6. Goodhand JR, Wahed M, Rampton DS. Management of stress in inflammatory bowel disease: a therapeutic option? *Expert Review of Gastroenterological Hepatology* 2009;3(6):661–79.

7. Knowles SR, Monshat K, Castle DJ. The efficacy and methodological challenges of psychotherapy for adults with inflammatory bowel disease: a review. *Inflammatory Bowel Diseases* 2013;19(12):2704–15.

8. Keefer L. Cognitive behaviour therapy and hypnotherapy in IBD. In: Knowles SR, Mikocka-Walus A (eds). *Psychological Aspects of Inflammatory Bowel Disease: A Biopsychosocial Approach.* London: Routledge; 2015. pp. 183–90.

9. Palsson OS. Hypnosis Treatment of Gastrointestinal Disorders: A Comprehensive Review of the Empirical Evidence. *American Journal of Clinical Hypnotherapy* 2015;58(2):134–58.

10. Harris R. *The Happiness Trap: How to Stop Struggling and Start Living: A Guide to ACT.* Wollombi, NSW: Exisle Publishing; 2008.

11. Csikszentmihaly M. *Flow.* New York: Harper Perennial Modern Classics; 2008.

Chapter 13

1. NHMRC. *NHMRC Information Paper: Evidence on the Effectiveness of Homeopathy for Treating Health Conditions.* Canberra: National Health and Medical Research Council; 2015.

2. Opheim R, Moum B. Complementary and alternative medicine in IBD. In: Knowles SR, Mikocka-Walus A (eds). *Psychological Aspects of Inflammatory Bowel Disease: A Biopsychosocial Approach.* London: Routledge; 2015. pp. 199–206.

3. Ji J, Lu Y, Liu H, Feng H, Zhang F, Wu L, et al. Acupuncture and moxibustion for inflammatory bowel diseases: a systematic review and meta-analysis of randomized controlled trials. Evidence-based Complementary and Alternative Medicine:

eCAM 2013;2013:158352.

4. Ng SC, Lam YT, Tsoi KK, Chan FK, Sung JJ, Wu JC. Systematic review: the efficacy of herbal therapy in inflammatory bowel disease. *Alimentary Pharmacology & Therapeutics* 2013;38(8):854–63.

5. Smith CA, Hay PP, Macpherson H. Acupuncture for depression. The Cochrane Database of Systematic Reviews 2010(1):CD004046.

6. Cramer H, Anheyer D, Lauche R, Dobos G. A systematic review of yoga for major depressive disorder. *Journal of Affective Disorders* 2017;213:70–7.

7. Yeung WF, Chung KF, Ng KY, Yu YM, Zhang SP, Ng BF, et al. Prescription of Chinese herbal medicine in pattern-based traditional Chinese medicine treatment for depression: a systematic review. Evidence-based Complementary and Alternative Medicine: eCAM 2015;2015:160189.

8. Manheimer E, Cheng K, Wieland LS, Min LS, Shen X, Berman BM, et al. Acupuncture for treatment of irritable bowel syndrome. *The Cochrane Database of Systematic Reviews* 2012(5):CD005111.

9. Schumann D, Anheyer D, Lauche R, Dobos G, Langhorst J, Cramer H. Effect of yoga in the therapy of irritable bowel syndrome: a systematic review. *Clinical Gastroenterology and Hepatology: The Official Clinical Practice Journal of the American Gastroenterological Association* 2016;14(12):1720–31.

10. Zhu JJ, Liu S, Su XL, Wang ZS, Guo Y, Li YJ, et al. Efficacy of Chinese herbal medicine for diarrhea-predominant irritable bowel syndrome: a meta-analysis of randomized, double-blind, placebo-controlled trials. Evidence-based Complementary and Alternative Medicine: eCAM 2016;2016:4071260.

Conclusion

1. The Lancet. A cure for Crohn's disease by 2032. *Lancet* 2017;389(10066):226.

Index

Also available...

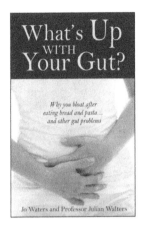

What's Up With Your Gut?
Why you bloat after eating bread and pasta... and other gut problems

By Jo Waters and Professor Julian Walters

What's Up With Your Gut? takes a practical look at the full range of gut problems, using a symptom-led approach so that sufferers can recognise what may have been troubling them for years and find solutions.

It then describes the range of solutions, both standard and alternative, emphasising the importance of what is eaten/ food intolerances and the impact of poor digestion on overall health. Whether you suffer cramping diarrhoea when you are stressed out, get constipated when you're on holiday or just feel fatigued by your grumbling guts, they show what the options are for diagnosis, symptom improvement and tackling the underlying causes.

www.hammersmithbooks.co.uk/product/your-gut/

Also available...

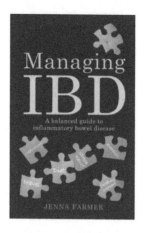

Managing IBD
A balanced guide to inflammatory bowel disease

By Jenna Farmer

**With IBD nurse specialist, Kaye Downes,
and counsellor/therapist, Sally Baker**

Jenna Farmer offers an holistic and positive guide to living
with IBD, combining conventional, nutritional, stress reduction
and other lifestyle approaches, drawing on her blogs, ebooks
and website www.abalancedbelly.co.uk. Throughout, the book
is 'illustrated' with case histories from Jenna's blog and other
contacts, and from her own experience of delayed diagnosis and
listening to her symptoms.

www.hammersmithbooks.co.uk/product/
managing-ibd-balanced-guide-inflammatory-bowel-disease/